NEUROANATOMY RESEARCH AT THE LEADING EDGE

NEW DEVELOPMENTS IN DOPAMINE RESEARCH

NEUROANATOMY RESEARCH AT THE LEADING EDGE

Additional books in this series can be found on Nova's website under the Series tab.

Additional e-books in this series can be found on Nova's website under the eBooks tab.

NEUROANATOMY RESEARCH AT THE LEADING EDGE

NEW DEVELOPMENTS IN DOPAMINE RESEARCH

GLEN HOPKINS

EDITOR

NOVA BIOMEDICAL

New York

Library of Congress Cataloging-in-Publication Data

ISBN: 978-1-63484-789-6

Library of Congress Control Number: 2016932181

Published by Nova Science Publishers, Inc. † New York

CONTENTS

PREFACE

Dopamine is an important neurotransmitter in human brain, and it is involved in many activities under physiological and pathological conditions of humans and mammals, especially in sports regulation, learning and memory, as well as drug addiction. Lack of dopamine can lead to a number of diseases such as schizophrenia, depression, and Parkinson's Disease. Thus, the studies of dopamine are of great importance in many disciplines such as neurophysiology, clinical medicine, and the pharmaceutical sciences. In recent years, more and more researchers have focused on the detection of dopamine and many different types of testing methods have emerged. Chapter One in this book reviews different kinds of electrodes used in the detection of dopamine and the stability, selectivity, sensitivity of those electrodes. Chapter Two presents a discussion about the modulation of the dopamine synthesis and release in the retina by light, clock genes and melatonin. Chapter Three summarizes the most recent findings on the role of central D_2, D_3 and D_4 receptors on erectile function and sexual behavior.

Chapter 1 – Dopamine is an important neurotransmitter in human brain, and it is involved in many activities under physiological and pathological conditions of humans and mammals, especially in the sports regulation, learning and memory, as well as drug addiction plays a key role. Lack of dopamine will lead to a number of important diseases such as schizophrenia, depression, Parkinson's disease, so the studies of dopamine are of great importance in many areas such as disciplines neurophysiology, clinical medicine, pharmaceutical science. In recent years, more and more researchers have focused on the detection of dopamine and many different types of testing methods have emerged. Among the detection methods, the electrochemical detection method due to its high selectivity, sensitivity and good stability turn into the ideal method for the detection of dopamine. In previous studies, scientists have made significant progress in the electrochemical detection of dopamine. But there are still many deficiencies in the electrochemical detection of dopamine and the innovation and development of this method eagerly. According to the different materials and preparation mechanisms of electrochemical sensors, different kinds of electrodes used in the detection of dopamine and the stability, selectivity, sensitivity of those electrodes is reviewed in this chapter. And the future direction of the electrochemical detection of dopamine is forecasted.

Chapter 2 – There is a vast literature about the dopamine importance in the retinal physiology and pathophysiology. Additionally, the vertebrate retina is a good model to study neurological diseases caused by disturbs in dopamine neurochemistry, since this tissue contains a complete dopaminergic system. The enzyme limiting of the velocity in the dopamine synthesis is the tyrosine hydroxylase (TH).

In the retina, TH is located in a subpopulation of the interneurons known as amacrine cells and interplexiform cells. Dopamine levels present a diurnal circadian behavior for the reason that they are modulated by light, clock genes and melatonin. The dopamine synthesis and release are inhibited by the nocturnal pineal hormone melatonin through a mechanism still devoid of the investigation. Melatonin is mainly produced by photoreceptors and melatonin membrane receptors are located in amacrine cells from retinas of all vertebrates studied, including humans. These receptors signalize mainly by Gi protein, however the melatonin pathway used in the modulation of the dopamine release does not include the inhibition of the cAMP levels, at least in chick retina development. This chapter presents a discussion about the modulation of the dopamine synthesis and release in the retina by light, clock genes and melatonin.

Chapter 3 – Among neurotransmitters involved in the control of erectile function and sexual behavior, dopamine is one of the most studied. Since the first pioneering studies done in the nineteen sixties, which revealed the facilitatory role of this neurotransmitter in sexual behavior, today it is well accepted that dopamine is deeply involved in both the anticipatory (appetitive and rewarding) and consummatory (penile erection and ejaculation) phases of sexual behavior. Dopamine influences sexual behavior by acting at the level of several brain areas (i.e., medial preoptic area, paraventricular nucleus of the hypothalamus and ventral tegmental area that contains the cell bodies of mesolimbic dopaminergic neurons projecting to the nucleus accumbens). The facilitation of sexual function by dopamine is mediated mainly by the stimulation of receptors of the D2 family (D_2, D_3 and D_4), with only a minor role for those of the D1 family (D_1 and D_5). In spite of the large amount of preclinical studies showing a facilitatory role of D_2-like receptors in sexual behavior, scarce success was obtained with classic D_2-like agonists (mainly apomorphine), especially when compared to that obtained with locally acting phosphodiesterase type V inhibitors, in the treatment of erectile dysfunction in humans. The discovery of selective D_4 receptor agonists able to induce penile erection with potency similar to that of classic mixed D_2 agonists in male rats has reopened the research aimed at the identification of dopamine agonists useful for the treatment of erectile dysfunction in humans. This review summarizes the most recent findings on the role of central D_2, D_3 and D_4 receptors on erectile function and sexual behavior. These studies suggest that D_4 receptors may represent a valuable therapeutic target for the therapy of erectile dysfunction.

In: New Developments in Dopamine Research ISBN: 978-1-63484-789-6
Editor: Glen Hopkins

Chapter 1

ELECTROCHEMICAL DETECTION OF DOPAMINE USING CARBON NANOMATERIAL BASED ELECTRODES

Hailin Cong[1,2,*], Bing Yu[1,2,†], Xiulan Zhang[1] and Shujing Yang[1]

[1]College of Material Science and Engineering,
Qingdao University, Qingdao 266071, China
[2]Laboratory for New Fiber Materials and Modern Textile,
Growing Base for State Key Laboratory, Qingdao University, China

ABSTRACT

Dopamine is an important neurotransmitter in human brain, and it is involved in many activities under physiological and pathological conditions of humans and mammals, especially in the sports regulation, learning and memory, as well as drug addiction plays a key role. Lack of dopamine will lead to a number of important diseases such as schizophrenia, depression, Parkinson's disease, so the studies of dopamine are of great importance in many areas such as disciplines neurophysiology, clinical medicine, pharmaceutical science. In recent years, more and more researchers have focused on the detection of dopamine and many different types of testing methods have emerged.

* Corresponding author: hailincong@yahoo.com; yubingqdu@163.com.
† E-mail: yubingqdu@yahoo.com.

Among the detection methods, the electrochemical detection method due to its high selectivity, sensitivity and good stability turn into the ideal method for the detection of dopamine. In previous studies, scientists have made significant progress in the electrochemical detection of dopamine. But there are still many deficiencies in the electrochemical detection of dopamine and the innovation and development of this method eagerly. According to the different materials and preparation mechanisms of electrochemical sensors, different kinds of electrodes used in the detection of dopamine and the stability, selectivity, sensitivity of those electrodes is reviewed in this chapter. And the future direction of the electrochemical detection of dopamine is forecasted.

Keywords: dopamine, modified electrode, graphene, single-walled carbon nanotubes, fullerene

1. Introduction

Dopamine (DA) is a natural catecholamine formed by the decarboxylation of 3, 4-dihydroxyphenylalanine, which belongs to the family of excitatory chemical neurotransmitters [1-3], and it is one of the important neurotransmitters that are widely distributed in the mammalian central nervous system for message transfer. It is mainly responsible for the reward sensation, and transmits the information of excitement and fun, at the same time, related to the addiction [4]. It is of great clinical importance to measure the DA level in extracellular fluid to monitor neurotransmission processes and diagnose Parkinson disease [5]. Therefore, it is of great importance to sensitively and selectively monitor DA not only for biomedical chemistry and neurochemistry research but also for diagnostic and pathological purpose. As we all know, dopamine (DA), uric acid (UA), and ascorbic acid (UA) are always coexisted in the extra cellular fluids of central nervous system and serum in mammals, which play very important roles in human metabolism [6, 7]. UA is a vital vitamin in human diet and very popular in foodstuffs for its antioxidant properties [8]. Thus, the UA concentration is much higher (100-1000 times) than that of DA in body fluids. Therefore, selective detection of DA and UA, and even their simultaneous detection in the presence of large amount of UA have received tremendous attention in biomedical chemistry, and diagnostic and pathological researches [9, 10], owing to their similar properties.

To date, several impressive techniques have demonstrated the feasibility for the assay of DA, including electrochemical [11–16], colorimetric [17–20], fluorescence spectrometry [21], liquid chromatography/electrospray tandem mass spectrometry [22], and high performance liquid chromatography methods [23]. Among these, electrochemical approaches haveattracted most attention because of their simplicity, low instrumental cost, and capability in real-time and even in vivo measurements. Although the electrochemical responses have been continuously improved, the development ofmore reliable andefficient sensors for sensitive analysis of DA still remains very challenging. Therefore, the choice of material is essential and important to construct sensors with excellent performance.

Graphene (GR) is a material that attracts more and more attention in many fields of electronics, optical, magnetic, biological medicine, catalysis, energy storage due to its special nanostructures and superior performance [24, 25]. It is also usually used in sensorapplications because of its large surface area and high electrocatalytic activity [26-29]. In recent years, some researchers used electrodes modified by graphene composites to determine DA, such as nitrogen doped graphene glassy carbon electrode (GCE), graphene/Pt GCE, gold nanoparticles-b-cyclodextrin/graphene GCE [30-32], and all of these modified electrodes have excellent experimental results. Diazoresin (DR), as a photosensitive polyelectrolyte, has been massively utilized in the self-assembly system to improve the stability of the self-assembled multilayer films via photo-crosslinking technique [33, 34]. For example, the unstable ionic linkage involved in the multilayers will convert to stable covalent bonds with exposure of the DR containing films to UV light.

The hardness of single-walled carbon nanotubes is the same as the diamond, but it also has good flexibility and can be stretched [35]. The conductivity ofsingle-walled carbon nanotubes is very good, and which is also the reason why the single-walled carbon nanotube can be applied in electrochemistry field. Because of its unique mechanical, electronic and chemical properties, C_{60} becomes a research focus gradually since the advent of it. The C_{60}-specific catalytic effect for electrode modification, in addition to be able to introduce its own physical and chemical properties of the electrode interface, but also due to the large surface area C_{60} effect, surface functional groups to carry more than produce certain substances on the electrochemical behavior [36].

Various self-assembly methodologies have achieved great diversity [37-39]. Diazoresin (DR), as a photosensitive polyelectrolyte, has been massively utilized in self-assembly systems to improve the stability of the self-assembled multilayer films via the photocrosslinking technique [33, 34, 40-42]. For example, the unstable ionic linkages involved in the multilayers will convert to stablecovalentbondswithexposureofthe DRcontainingfilms to UV light. In this article, we applied the self-assembly method combined with the photocrosslinking technique to the preparation of DR/GR modified Au electrodes, DR/SWNT modified Au electrodes, Carboxyl-C_{60} ModifiedElectrodes, and investigated the electrochemical behavior of DA on the electrodes by the methods of cyclic voltammeter (CV) and differential pulse voltammeter (DPV).

2.DIAZORESIN/GARPHENEMODIFIED ELECTRODES

2.1. Fabrication of DR/GR ModifiedElectrodes

The schematic fabrication process was illustrated in Figure 1.

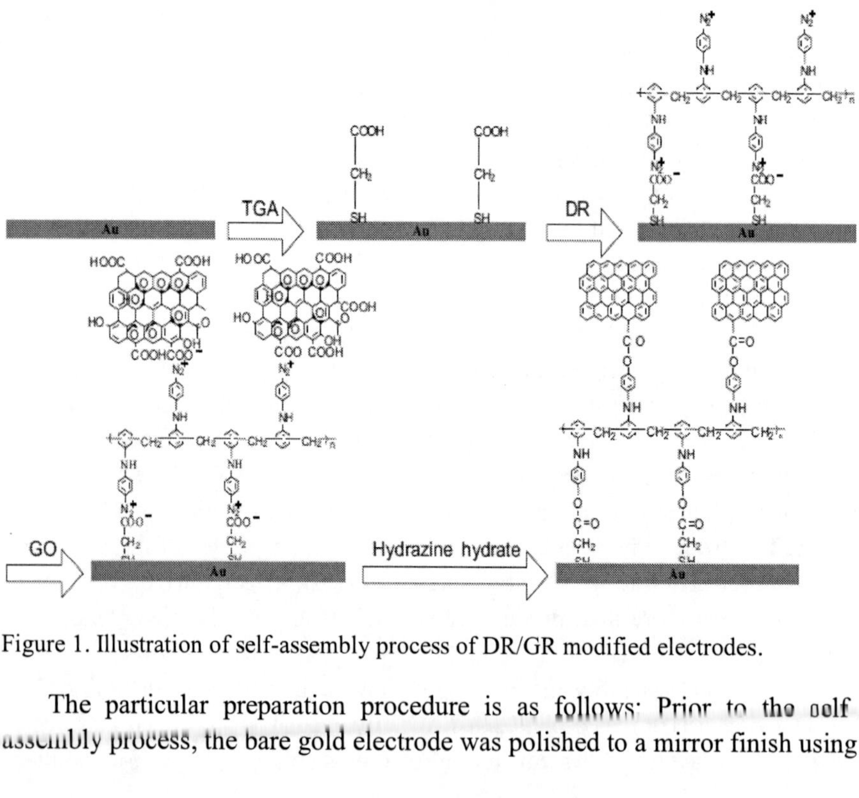

Figure 1. Illustration of self-assembly process of DR/GR modified electrodes.

The particular preparation procedure is as follows: Prior to the self-assembly process, the bare gold electrode was polished to a mirror finish using aqueous alumina (particle size 0.05 μm) slurry, and rinsed with deionized water. The treated gold electrode was immersed in aqueous solution of 0.1MTGA at room temperature for 3 hours. And then, the electrode was rinsed by anhydrous alcohol and deionized water to remove non-specific adsorption TGA. After N2 drying, the electrode was alternately immersed in aqueous polycation DR solution (0.05 M) and aqueous graphene oxide dispersion (0.05 M) for 5 min and 10 min, respectively. The electrode was then rinsed thoroughly with deionized water and dried with N2 to complete the assembly process. Finally, the modified electrode was exposed to 0.05 M hydrazine hydrate for 2 h to finish the whole fabrication process.

2.2. DR/GR Modified Electrodes Performance

After detecting the behaviors of the dopamine by this modified electrode using electrochemical methods and concluded that: Compared to bare Au electrodes, the DR/GR modified electrodes show well-defined and resolved voltammetric responses for the direct oxidation of DA. The oxidation peak current at the modified electrode is much higher than that of the bare electrode, which indicates that the DR/GR modified electrode is an effective electro catalyst for the oxidation of DA. The same conclusion is also shown in Figure 2.

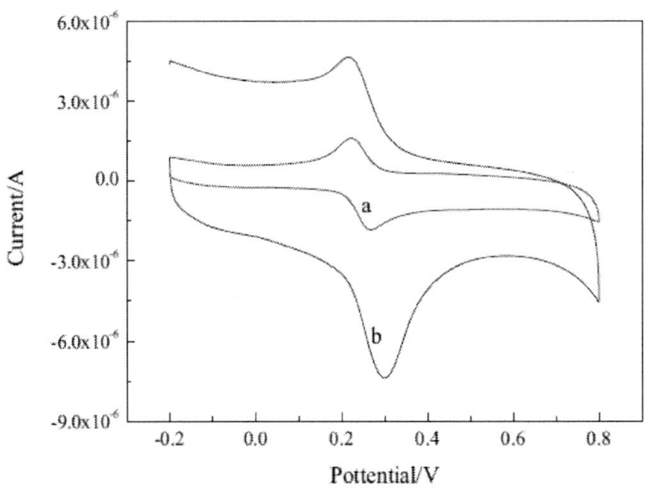

Figure 2. CV responses at the bare Au (a) and DR/GR modified electrodes (b) in 0.1 M PBS (pH6.0) containing 20 μM DA. Scan rate: 50 mV/s.

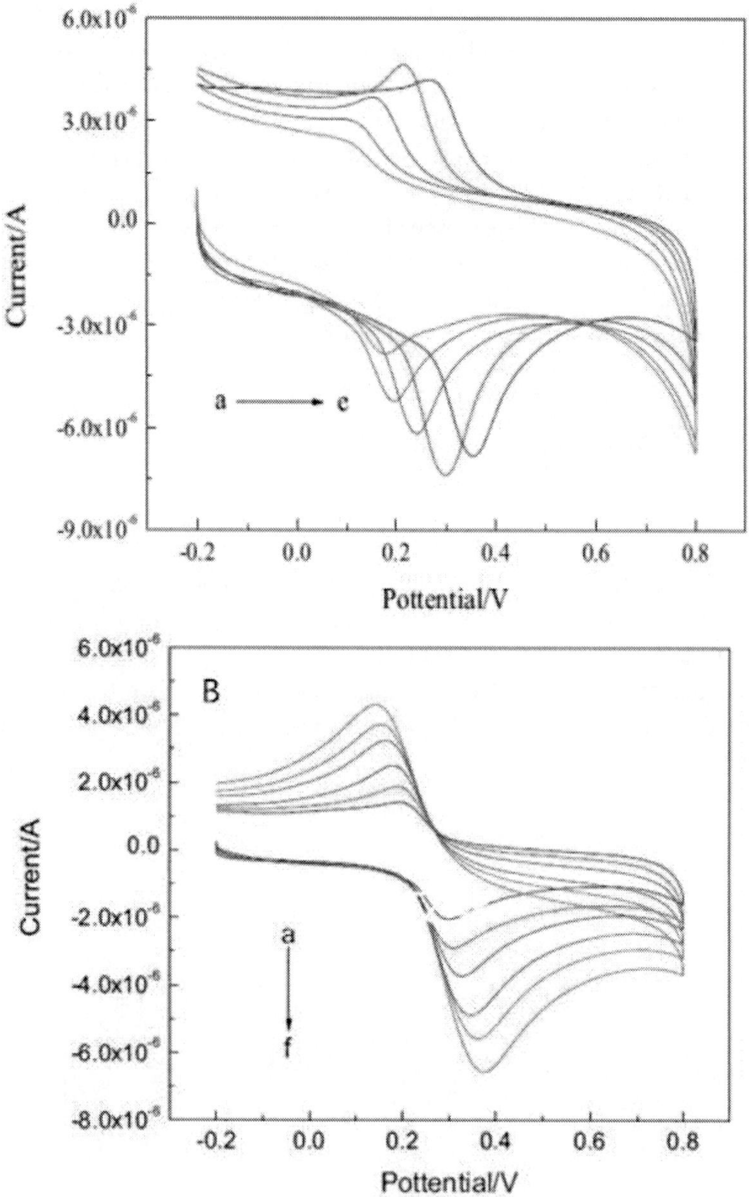

Figure 3. (Continued).

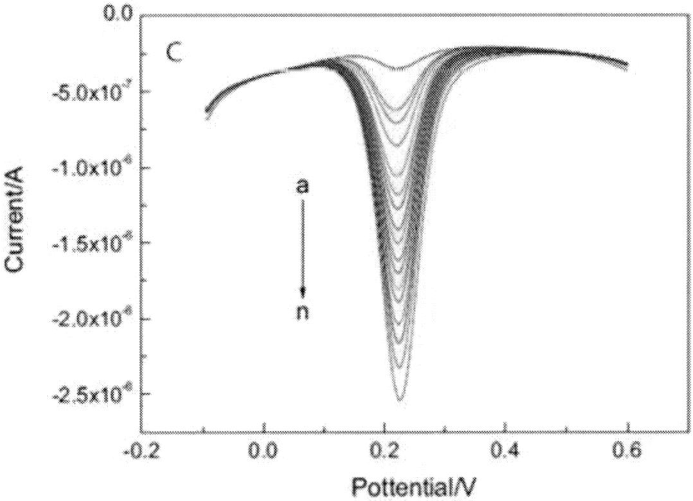

Figure 3. A. CV responses of 20 μM DA on DR/GR modified electrodes in 0.1 M PBS at different pH values (a–e: 9.0, 8.0, 7.0, 6.0, and 5.0, respectively); B. Effect of concentrations on the electro-oxidation of DA: (A) CV responses at DR/GR modified electrodes in pH 6.0 PBS of different DA concentrations (a–f: 2, 6, 10, 14, 18 and 22 μM, respectively). Scan rate: 50 mV/s.

Continue to use the modified electrode in different conditions detected electrochemical behavior of dopamine, we can also find more effective conclusions. As shown in Figure 3A, the effect of pH on the electrochemical behaviors of 20 μM DA at the DR/GR Au is carefully investigated by CV in a range from pH 5.0 to pH 9.0 in 0.1 mM PBS. It is apparent that the highest peak currents are obtained at pH 6.0. Therefore, pH 6.0 is chosen for the subsequent analytical experiments. And according to Figure 3B, with the concentration of DA increased from 2 to 22 μM, the anodic peak was becoming higher and higher. The DPV responses of different concentration of DA on DR/GR modified electrodes were recorded and shown in Figure 3C, from which we can see that the peak currents are proportional to DA concentration in the range of 1–80 μM with a detection limit of 2.8×10^{-9} M (S/N = 3). These findings more favorable proved that the electrochemical behavior of detecting dopamine by using this modified electrode has improved significantly.

The stability of the DR/GR modified electrode is evaluated. After one-week storage at room temperature, 97.1% of the initial current signal was obtained and after two-week storage, 93.1% signal remained, indicating that the prepared electrode had excellent long-term stability. Meanwhile, the reproducibility of this modified electrode is investigated. When five modified electrodes from the same fabrication procedure are prepared and used for the DA determination, the RSD is 4.1%. These results indicate that the modified electrodes have good detecting and fabrication reproducibility, and excellent long-term stability.

2.3. Conclusion

The self-assembly method combined with photo-crosslinking technique was applied to the preparation of DR/GR modified Au electrodes successfully. The electrochemical behavior of DA on the modified electrodes was investigated by CV and DPV methods. The modified electrodes showed very high electrocatalytic activity towards DA oxidation with a significant enhancement in peak current. A sensitive DPV response to DA concentration from 1 to 80 μM was achieved. Additionally, the electrodes exhibited very good stability and reproducibility for the electrochemical determination of DA.

3. Diazoresin/Single-WalledCarbon Nanotube Modified Electrodes

3.1. Fabrication of DR/SWNT Modified Electrodes

The fabrication of DR/SWNT modified electrodes as shown in Figure 4: Prior to the self-assembly process, the bare gold electrode was polished to a mirror finish using aqueous alumina (particle size 0.05 mm) slurry, and rinsed with deionized water. The treated gold electrode was immersed in an aqueous solution of 0.1 mol/L thioglycollic acid (TGA) at room temperature for 3 h. And then, the electrode was rinsed by anhydrous alcohol and deionized water to remove non-specifically adsorbed TGA. After N2 drying, the electrode was alternately immersed in an aqueous polycation DR solution (0.05 mol/L) and an aqueous COOH-SWNT dispersion (0.05 mol/L) for 5 min and 10 min, respectively. The electrode was then rinsed thoroughly with deionized water and dried with N2 to complete the assembly process. Finally, the modified electrode was exposed to UV light from a medium-pressure mercury lamp with an intensity of 12 mW/cm^2 at 365 nm for 30 s to finish the whole fabrication process.

3.2. Electrochemical Behaviors of Dopamine at the DR/SWNT Electrodes

The electrocatalytic activity of the DR/SWNT modified electrodes toward the oxidation of DA is characterized by cyclic voltammetry (CV) ranging from 0.1 V to 0.6 V. The CV responses of 2 mmol/L DA in 0.1 mol/L PBS (pH 6.0) at the bare and DR/SWNT modified electrodes are shown in Figure 5. Compared to bare Au electrodes, the DR/SWNT modified electrodes show well-defined and resolved voltammetric responses for the direct oxidation of DA. The oxidation peak current at the modified electrode is much higher than that of the bare electrode, which indicates that the DR/ SWNT modified electrode is an effective electrocatalyst for the oxidation of DA.

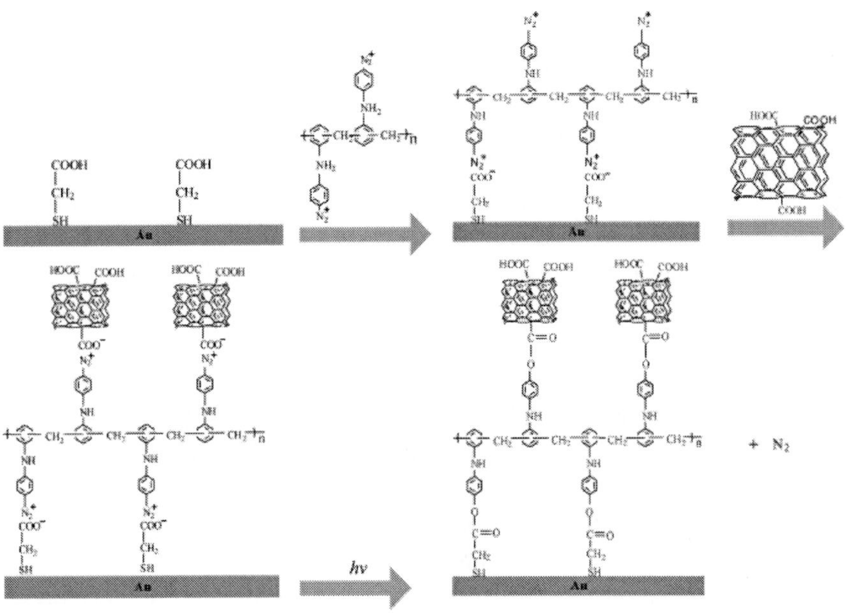

Figure 4. Illustration of self-assembly process of DR/SWNT modified electrodes.

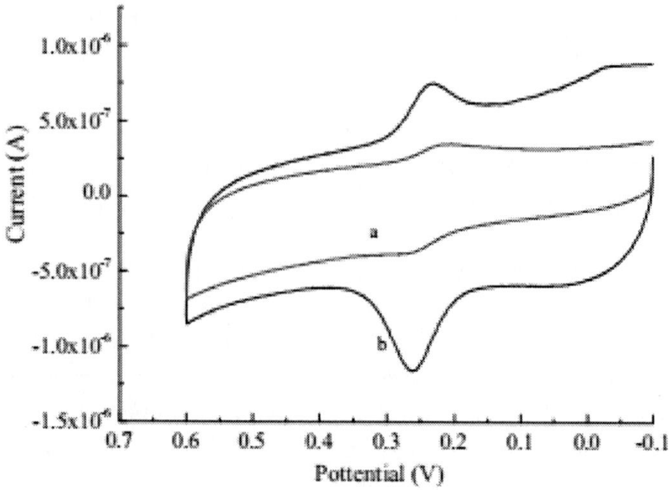

Figure 5. CV responses at the bare Au (a) and DR/SWNT modified electrodes (b) in 0.1 mol/L PBS (pH 6.0) containing 2 mmol/L DA. Scan rate: 50 mV/s.

Proton is always involved in the electrochemical reactions of organic compounds and exerts significant impact on the reaction rate. Therefore, the effect of pH is investigated by the CV method in 0.1 mol/L PBS over the range from pH 5.0 to 8.0. Figure 6A shows the CV results in 0.1 mol/L PBS containing 20 mmol/L of DA at different pH values. We can see that the electro-oxidation behavior of DA isdependent on the pH value of the solution. The peak potential for oxidation of DA shifts to more positive potentials with the changes of the pH of the solutions from alkaline to acidic values. The experiment is performed with the CV method in 0.1 mol/L PBS (pH 6.0). As shown in Figure 6B, with the concentration of DA increased from 1 mmol/L to 40 mmol/L, the anodic peak grew proportionally. Figure 6C presents the effect of scan rate on the electrochemical behaviors of 20 mmol/L DA in 0.1 mol/L PBS (pH 6.0) at the DR/ SWNT modified electrodes. From this picture, we can see that the oxidation peak currents of DA increase with increasing scan rates. It is indicated that the electrochemical redox behavior of DA at the modified electrodes surface is an adsorption-controlled process.

As shown in Figure 7A, the DPV method is used for the determination of DA in the presence of 10 mmol/L UA. The voltammograms of solutions with different concentrations of DA are. The peak currents are proportional to DA concentrations in the range of 2–80 mmol/L with a detection limit of 2.1×10^{-9} mol/L (S/N = 3). The DPV method is used for the determination of DA in the presence of 10 mmol/L AA. The voltammograms of solutions with different concentrations of DA are shown in Figure 7B. The peak currents are proportional to DA concentrations in the range of 2–100 mmol/L with a detection limit of 2.5×10^{-9}mol/L (S/N = 3).

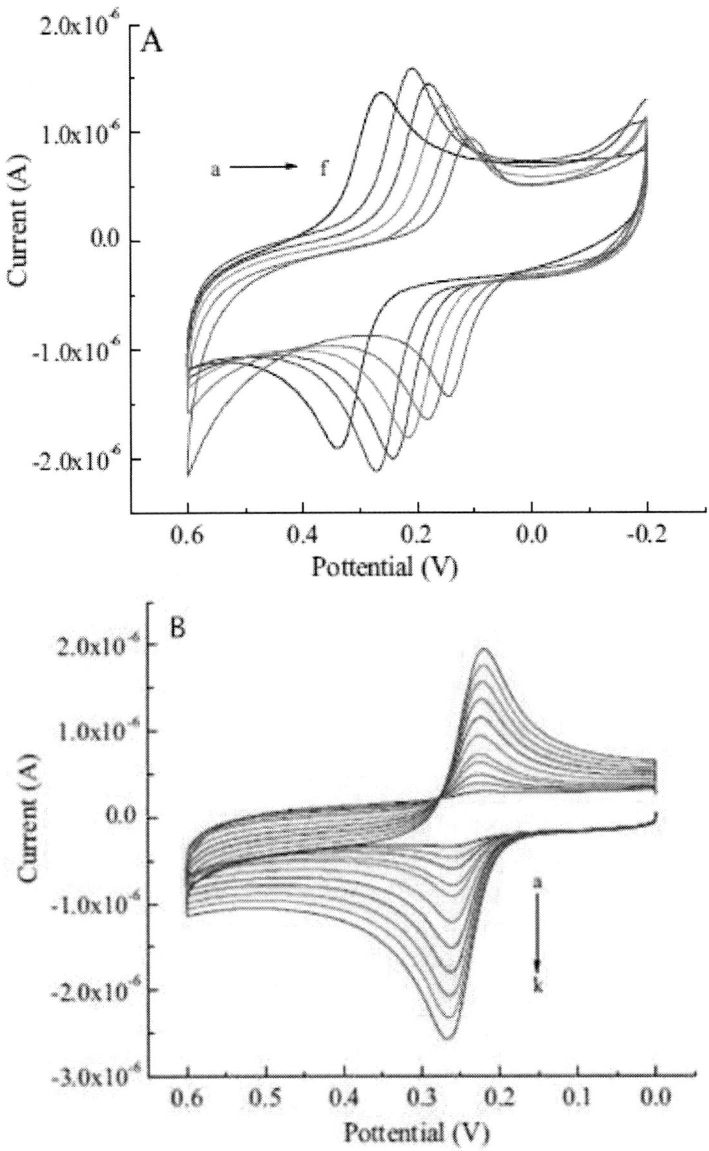

Figure 6. (Continued).

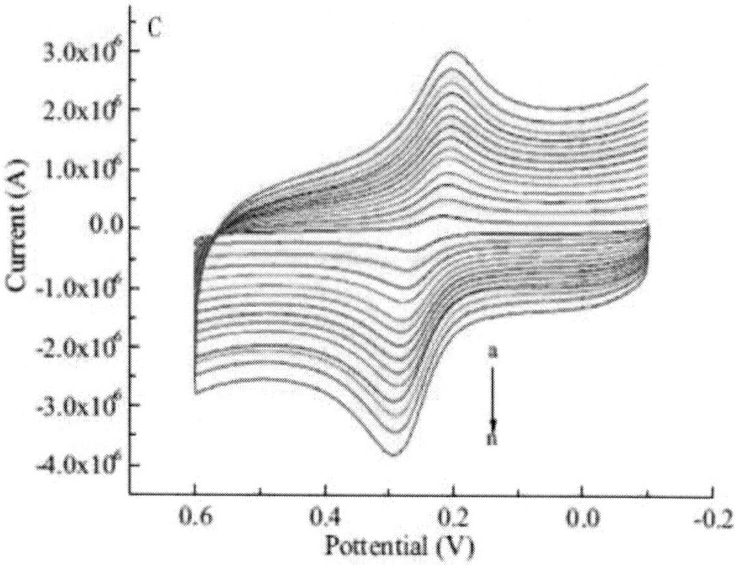

Figure 6. (A) Effect of pH on the electro-oxidation of DA:CV responses of 20 mmol/L DA on DR/SWNT modified electrodes in 0.1 mol/L PBS at different pH values (a–f: 5.0, 6.0, 6.5, 7.0, 7.5, and 8.0, respectively); Scan rate: 50 mV/s. (B)Effect of concentrations on the electro-oxidation of DA: CV responses at DR/SWNT modified electrodes in pH 6.0 PBS of different DA concentrations (a–f: 1, 3, 5, 8, 10, 15, 20, 25, 30, 35, and 40 mmol/L, respectively). Scan rate: 50 mV/s. (C) Effect of scan rate on the electro-oxidation of DA: CV responses of 20 mmol/L DA on DR/SWNT modified electrodes in pH 6.0 PBS at various scan rates (a–n: 10.0, 30.0, 50.0, 70.0, 90.0, 110.0, 130.0, 150.0, 170.0, 190.0, 210.0, 230.0, 260.0, 280.0, and 300.0 mV/s, respectively).

In order to prove that the modified electrode is still applicable to the actual application, our recent experiments demonstrate that the modified electrodes not only can determine DA in the presence of main interferences such as UA and AA, but also can determine DAHCl in the real samples of dopamine hydrochloride injection. As shown in Figure 8, the peak currents are proportional to DAHCl concentration in the range of 0.01–100 mmol/L. Therefore, the DR/SWNT modified electrode showed high sensitivity and selectivity for detection of DAHCl in the real sample of DHI. The recovery test performed indicated that the DR/SWNT modified electrodes had very good recovery rates for the direct electrochemical determination of DAHCl in the real samples.

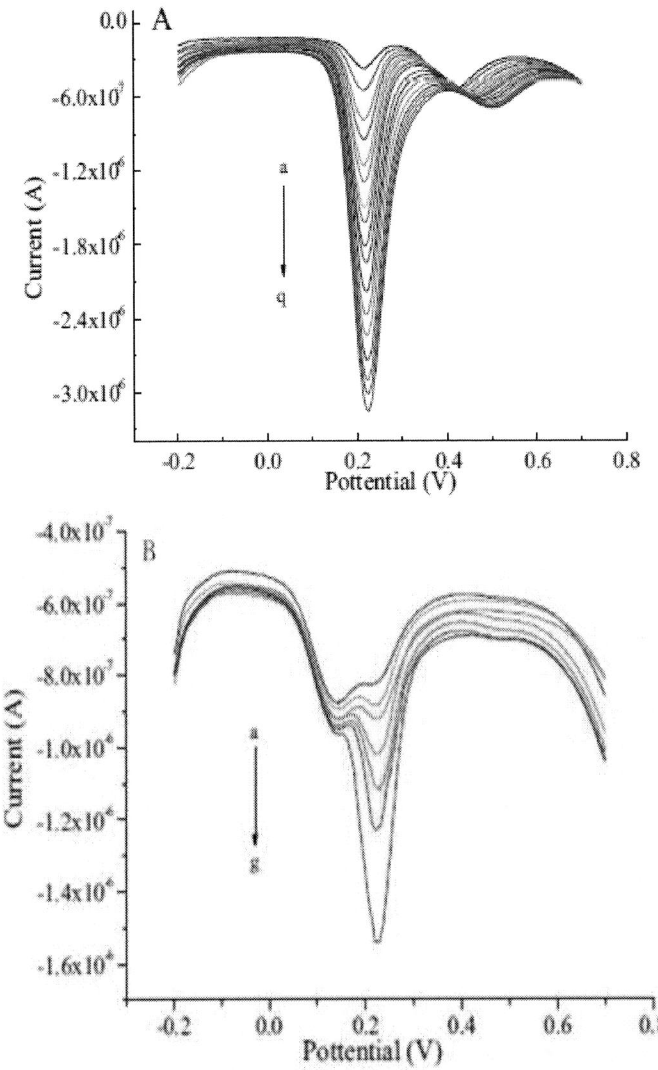

Figure 7. (A) Selective detection of DA in the presence of UA. DPV responses at DR/SWNT modified electrodes in 0.1 mol/L PBS (pH 6.0) containing 10 mmol/L of UA and different concentrations of DA from 2 mmol/L to 120 mmol/L (a–q: 2, 6, 12, 16, 22, 26, 32, 36, 42, 46, 52, 60, 70, 80, 90, 100, 110 and 120 mmol/L, respectively); (B)Selective detection of DA in the presence of AA. DPV responses at DR/SWNT modified electrodes in 0.1 mol/L PBS (pH 6.0) containing 10 mmol/L of AA and different concentrations of DA from 2 mmol/L to 100 mmol/L (a–g: 2, 8, 15, 25, 40, 55 and 100 mmol/L, respectively). Scan rate: 50 mV/s.

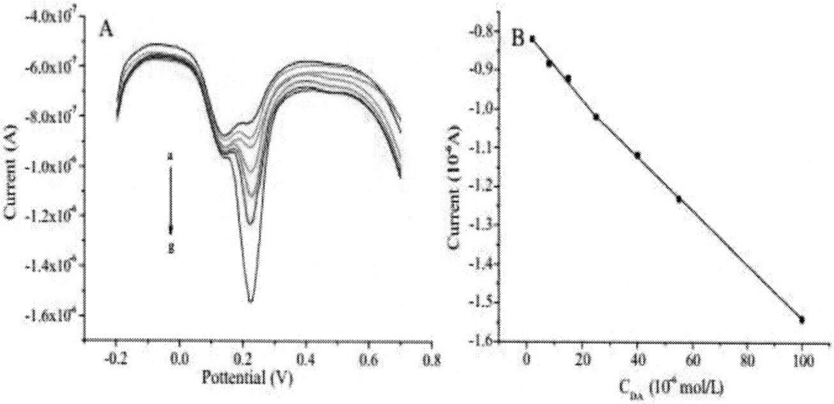

Figure 8.Selective detection of DA-HCl in real sample of dopamine hydrochloride injection. (A) DPV responses at DR/SWNT modified electrodes in 0.1 mol/L PBS (pH 6.0) containing different concentrations of DA-HClfrom 0.01 mmol/L to 100 mmol/L (a–g: 0.01, 2, 4, 10, 20, 40 and 100 mmol/L, respectively). Scan rate: 50 mV/s. (B) Relationship between the oxidation peaks current versus concentration of DAHCl.

The stability of the DR/SWNT modified electrodes is evaluated. After one-week storage at room temperature, 98.2% of the initial current signal was retained, and after two-week storage, 97.2% signal remained, indicating that the prepared electrodes have excellent long-term stability. Meanwhile, the reproducibility of these modified electrodes is investigated. When five modified electrodes from the same fabrication procedure are prepared and used for the DA determination, the RSD is 3.4%. These results indicate that the modified electrodes have good detecting and fabrication reproducibility.

3.3. Conclusion

The self-assembly method combined with the photocrosslinking technique was applied to the preparation of DR/ SWNT modified Au electrodes successfully. The electrochemical behavior of DA on the modified electrodes was investigated by the CV and DPV methods. The modified electrodes exhibited good stability and reproducibility for the electrochemical determination of DA. Moreover, the modified electrodes showed very high electrocatalytic activity toward DA oxidation with a significant enhancement in peak current. Under the optimal conditions, a linear CV response to DA concentrations from 1 mmol/L to 40 mmol/L was observed, and the detection limit of DA was 2.1××10^{-3}mmol/L via the DPV method in the presence of 10 mmol/L of UA or 2.5×10^{-3}mmol/L via the DPV method in the presence of 10 mmol/L of AA. Additionally, the DR/SWNT modified electrodes showed high sensitivity and selectivity for detection of DA-HCl in the real samples of dopamine hydrochloride injection. The advantage of this modified electrode is that photosensitive DR as a polyelectrolyte is applied to the layer-by-layer self-assembly modification process, and after UV photocrosslinking, the unstable ionic linkages involved in the self-assembled multilayers convert to stable covalent bonds, which makes the modified electrodes have better stability and fabrication reproducibility.

4. CARBOXYL-C_{60}MODIFIED ELECTRODES PERFORMANCE

4.1. Fabrication of Carboxyl-C_{60} Modified Electrodes

The fullerene were suspended in a 3M HNO_3 solution and kept them for about 10 h in reflux until the evolution of NO_2 vapors subsided. After this treatment, the solid product was separated by centrifuge and then washed successively using deionized water. 3M HCl, and deionized water. After dried under vacuum at 50°C, a black powder was obtained. The gold electrode was polished successively using 0.3 μm and 0.5 μm Al_2O_3 powder and rinsed thoroughly with ethanol and water each for 5 min, and then dried at room temperature. 5 mg Carboxyl-C_{60} was dispersed in deionized water by ultrasonication. A 5μL C_{60} suspension was then pipetted onto the pretreated gold electrode surface and dried at room temperature.

4.2. Electrochemical Behaviors of Dopamine at the Carboxyl-C_{60} Modified Electrode

Figure 2 shows the CVs of the Carboxyl-C_{60} modified electrodes and bare Au electrodes in 0.1 M PBS (pH 6.0) containing 5 μM DA and 5 μM UA. Evidently, two distinct anodic peaks is found for the Carboxyl-C_{60} modified electrodes, which are attributed to the oxidation of DA and UA, respectively, as above demonstrated. These results indicate that the Carboxyl-C_{60} which has good electrocatalytic activity, conductivity and large specific surface area modified electrodes can improve the redox of the probe, which is attributed to its high electric conductivity.

Simultaneous detection of DA and UA was performed on the Carboxyl-C_{60} modified electrodes in 0.1 M PBS containing 10 μM UA. As illustrated in Figure 10A with the increase of the DA concentrations in the presence of 10 μM UA, the anodic peak currents of DAare linearly increased ranging from 5.0 to 45 μM. Similar trend are observed by increasing the UA concentrations from 10.0 to 90 μM (Figure 10B) in the solution containing 10 μM DA. The results obtained from Figure 3. Indicating that simultaneous determination of DA and UA can be selectively and sensitively on the Carboxyl- C_{60} modified electrodes.

In order to understand the feasibility in practical application, the Carboxyl-C_{60} modified electrode was used to determine DA and UA in real human urine samples which were diluted with 0.1 M PBS (pH 6.0). DPV curves obtained in urine samples and the determination of UA (and DA) are reported with several additions of analyte in Figure 11. From Figure 11 we can see that the electrode is sensitive enough, which are in close agreement with the values of the previous report [21]. The good recoveries of the mixture samples containing both DA and UA suggest that the Carboxyl-C_{60} modified electrode is of practical utilization for the determination of DA and UA.

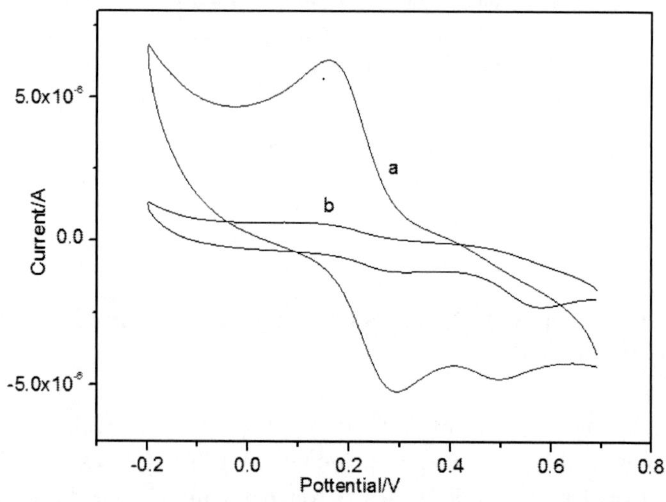

Figure 9. CV responses at Carboxyl- C_{60} modified electrodes (a) and the bare Au (b) containing 5 μM DA and 5 μM UA in 0.1 M PBS (pH 6.0). Scan rate: 50 mV/s.

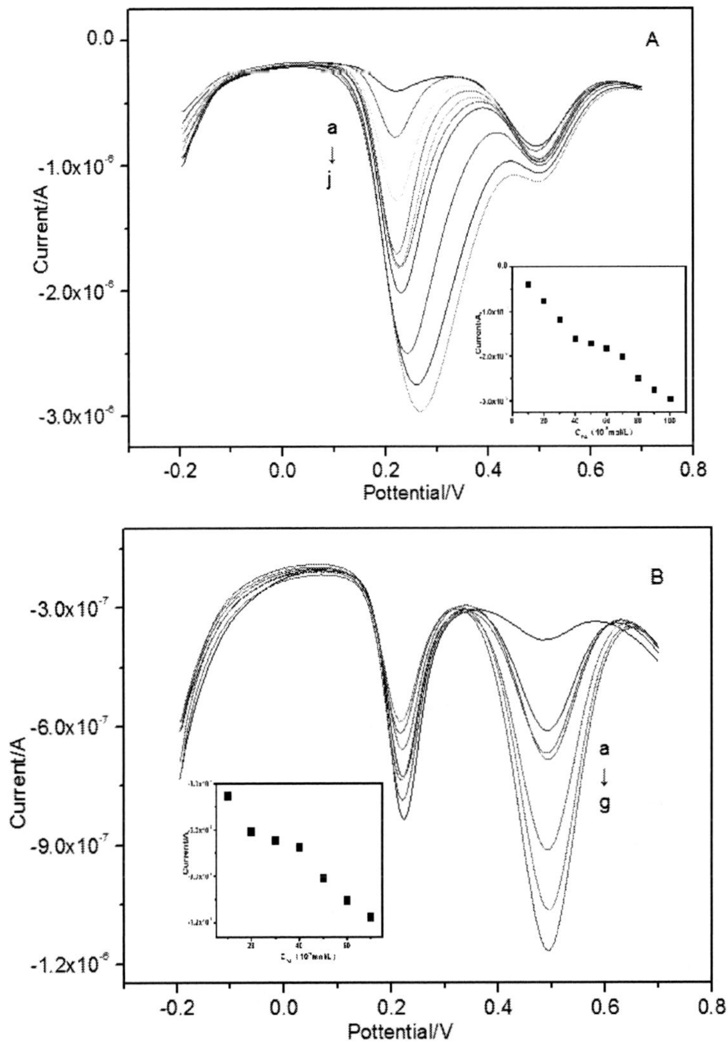

Figure 10. (A) DPV responses at Carboxyl- C_{60} modified electrodes in 0.1 M PBS (pH 6.0) containing 10 μM UA and different concentrations of DA from 5 μM to 45 μM (a-j: 5, 10, 15, 20, 25, 30, 35, 40 and 45 μM, respectively). (B) DPV of Carboxyl- C_{60} modified electrodes in 0.1 M PBS (pH 6.0) containing 10 μM DA and different concentrations of UA from 20 μM to 80 μM (a-g: 20, 30, 40, 50, 60, 70 and 80 μM, respectively). Scan rate: 50 mV/s.

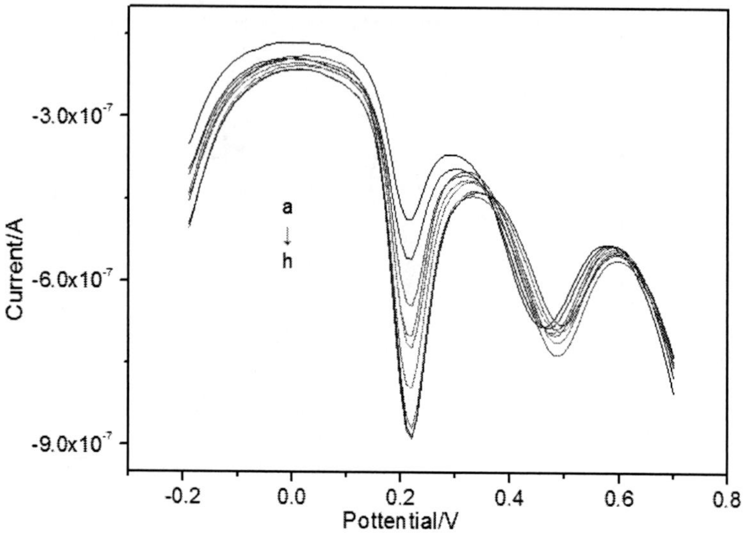

Figure 11. DPV of urine samples containing10 μM UA and different concentrations of DA from 5 μM to 40 μM (a-h: 5, 10, 15, 20, 15, 20, 25, 30, 35 and 40 μM, respectively). Scan rate: 50 mV/s.

Reproducibility and stability is an important standard to examine the electrochemical sensors. Prepared five electrodes in the same time, after repeating ten times in the same concentration of DA, the relative deviation of the current response is 5.4%. These results indicated that the modified electrodes have good detecting and fabrication reproducibility. Meanwhile, the stability of these modified electrodes is investigated. After one-week storage at room temperature, 97.6% of the initial current signal is obtained, and after two-weekstorage, 96.8% signal is remained, indicating that prepared electrodes have excellent longterm stability.

4.3. Conclusion

The use of Carboxyl-C60 modified electrodes can improve the sensitivity ofthe sensor significantly. And we successfully prepared electrochemical sensor in detectionof DA. This modified electrode in detection of DA showed good linearity in the rangeof $5.0 \times 10^{-7} \sim 6.0 \times 10^{-5}\mu$mol/L, and the detection limit of DA is $4.0 \times 10^{-8}\mu$mol/L. Thissensor for detecting of DA has good sensitivity and selectivity, and successfully used fordetection of the actual sample.

CONCLUSION

In thiswork, a variety of carbonmaterialsmodifiedelectrodeswereprepared and applied in the electrochemicaldetection of dopamine successfully. Compared with unmodified electrodes, the modified electrodesexihibted good electrochemical behavior.When using the modified electrodes to detect dopamine, the behavior of the modified electrodes have a higher sensitivity, better selectivity and good stability. The modiifed electrodes is cheap and can detect dopamine in more complex conditions. And provide a more affordable method to detect dopamine by electrochemical methods. But there are still many deficiencies in the electrochemical detection of dopamine and the innovation and development of this method eargely. More researches should be carried on the electrochemical detection of dopamine and overcome the drawbacks of the current detection methods and promote the development of electrochemical detection of dopamine.

ACKNOWLEDGMENTS

This work is financially supported by the Natural Science Foundation of China (21375069, 21404065, 21574072), the Natural Science Foundation for Distinguished Young Scientists of Shandong Province (JQ201403), the Project of Shandong Province Higher Educational Science and Technology Program (J15LC20), the Graduate Education Innovation Project of Shandong Province (SDYY14028), the Scientific Research Foundation for the Returned Overseas Chinese Scholars of State Education Ministry (20111568), the Science and Technology Program of Qingdao (1314159jch) and the Postdoctoral Scientific Research Foundation of Qingdao.

REFERENCES

[1] Wightman, R. M., May, L. J. & Michael, A. C.(1988). Detection of dopamine dynamics in the brain. *Anal. Chem.*, *60*, 769A–779A.

[2] Yu, B., Yuan, H., Yang, Y.Y., Cong, H.L., Hao, T.Z., Xu, X.D., Zhang, X.L., Yang, S.J. & Zhang, L.X. (2014). Detection of dopamine using self-assembled diazoresin/single-walledcarbon nanotube modified electrodes. *Chin. Chem. Lett.*, *25*, 523-528.

[3] Yang, Y.Y., Yu, B., Cong, H.L., Hao, T.Z., Lu, J., Zhang, J.D., Yuan, H.& Zhang, L.X. (2014). Determination of dopamine using self-assembled diazoresin/graphene modified electrodes. *Integr.Ferroelectr.*, *154*, 36-42.

[4] Han, D. X., Han, T. T., Shan, C. S., Ivaska, A. & Niu, L. (2010). Simultaneous determination of ascorbic acid, dopamine and uricacid with chitosan-graphene modified electrode. *Electroanalysis*, *22*, 2001–2008.

[5] Damier, P., Hirsch, E. C., Aqid, Y. & Graybiel, A. M. (1999). The substantianigra of the human brain II. Patterns of loss of dopamine-containing neurons in Parkinson's disease. *Brain*, *122*, 1437–1448.

[6] Balamurugan, A. & Chen, S.M. (2007). Poly(3,4-ethylene dioxythiophene-co-(5-amino-2-naphthalenesulfonicacid))(PEDOT-PANS) film modified glassy carbon electrode for selective detection of dopamine in the presence of ascorbic acid and uric acid. *Anal. Chim. Acta.*, *596*, 92-96.

[7] Yang, L., Liu, D., Huang, J. S. & You, T. Y. (2014). Simultaneous determination of dopamine, ascorbic acid and uric acid at electrochemically reduced graphene oxide modified electrode. *Sens. Actuators B.*, *193*, 166-172.

[8] Bruce, F., Culleton, M. D., Martin, G., Larson, ScD., William, B., Kannel, M. D. & Daniel Levy, M. D. (1999). Serum uric acid and risk for cardiovascular disease and death: The Framingham heart study. *Ann Intern Med.*, *131*, 7-13.

[9] Sun, C. L., Lee, H. H., Yang, J. M. & Wu, C.C. (2011). The simultaneous electrochemical detection of ascorbic acid, dopamine, and uric acid using graphene/size-selected Ptnanocomposites. *Biosens. Bioelectron.*, *26*, 3450–3454.

[10] Chih, Y. K. & Yang, M. C. (2013). A 2, 2-azino-bis (3-ethylbenzthiazoline-6-sulfonic acid)-immobilized electrode for the

simultaneous detection of dopamine and uric acid in the presence of ascorbic acid. *Bioelectrochemistry.*, *91*, 44–47.

[11] Chandra, U., Swamy, B. E. K. & Gilbert, O. (2010). Poly (amaranth) film based sensor for resolution of dopamine in the presence of uric acid: a voltammetric study. *Chin. Chem. Lett.*, *21*, 1490–1492.

[12] Song, W., Chen, Y., Xu, J. & Tian, D. B. (2010). A selectivevoltammetric detection for dopamineusing poly (gallic acid) film modified electrode, *Chin. Chem. Lett.*, *21*, 349–352.

[13] Poliakov, A. E., Dumshakova, A. V., Muginova, S. V. & Shekhovtsova, T. N. (2011). A peroxidasebased method for thedetermination of dopamine, adrenaline, and a-methyldopa in the presence of thyroid hormones in pharmaceutical forms. *Talanta*, *84*, 710–716.

[14] Liu, S., Yan, J., He, G.W., Zhong, D.D., Chen, J. X., Shi, L.Y., Zhou, X.M. & Jiang, H. J.(2012). Layer-by-layer assembled multilayer films of reduced graphene oxide/gold nanoparticles for the electrochemical detection of dopamine. *J. Electroanal. Chem.*, *672*, 40–44.

[15] Sheng, Z. H., Zheng, X. Q., Xu, J. Y., Bao, J., Wang, F.B. & Xia, X. H. (2012). Electrochemical sensor based on nitrogen doped graphene: simultaneous determination of ascorbic acid, dopamine and uric acid. *Biosens. Bioelectron.*, *34*, 125–131.

[16] Farjami, E., Campos, R., Nielsen, J. S., Gothelfet, K. V., Kjems, J. & Ferapontova,E. E. (2013). RNA aptamer-based electrochemical biosensor for selective and label-free analysis of dopamine. *Anal. Chem.*,*85*, 121–128.

[17] Kong, B., Zhu, A., Luo, Y., Tian, Y., Yu, T.T. & Shi, G.Y. (2011). Sensitive and selective colorimetric visualization ofcerebral dopamine based on double molecular recognition. *Angew. Chem. Int. Ed.*, *50*, 1837–1840.

[18] Su, H., Sun, B., Chen, L., Xu, Z. & Ai, S. (2012). Colorimetric sensing of dopamine based on theaggregation of gold nanoparticles induced by copper ions. *Anal. Methods*, *4*, 3981–3986.

[19] Liu, J. M., Wang, X. X., Cui, M. L., Lin, L.P., Jiang, S.L., Jiao, L. & Zhang, L. H. (2013). A promising non-aggregation colorimetric sensor of AuNRs-Ag^+ for determination of dopamine.*Sens. Actuators B.*, *176*, 97–102.

[20] Feng, J. J., Guo, H., Li, Y. F., Wang, Y. H., Chen, W. Y. & Wang, A. J. (2013). Single molecular functionalized gold nanoparticles for hydrogen-bonding recognition and colorimetric detection of dopamine

with high sensitivity and selectivity. *ACS Appl. Mater. Interfaces.*, *5*, 1226–1231.

[21] Li, S. S., Wu, H. L., Liu, Y. J., Gu, H. W. & Yu, R. Q. (2013). Simultaneous determination of tyrosine and dopamine in urine samples using excitation–emission matrix fluorescence coupled with second-order calibration. *Chin. Chem. Lett.*, *24*, 239–242.

[22] El-Beqqali, A., Kussak, A. & Abdel-Rehim, M. (2007). Determination of dopamine and serotonine in human urine samples utilizing microextraction online with liquidchromatography/electrospray tandem mass spectrometry. *J. Sep. Sci.*, *30*, 421–424.

[23] Rao, P. S., Rujikarn, N., Luber, J. M. & Tyras, D. H. (1989). A specific sensitive HPLC method for determination of plasma dopamine. *Chromatographia.*, *28*, 307–310.

[24] Novoselov, K. S., Geim, A. K., Morozov, S. V., Jiang, D., Zhang, Y., Dubonos, S. V., Grigorieva, I. V. & Firsov, A.A. (2004). Electric field effect in atomically thin carbon films. *Science.*, *306*, 666–669.

[25] Novoselov, K. S., Geim, A. K, Morozov, S. V., Jang, D., Katsnelson, M.I., Grigorieva, I.V., Dubonos, S. V. & Firsov, A.A. (2005). Two-dimensional gas of massless Dirac fermions in grapheme. *Nature.*, *438*, 197–200.

[26] Song, Y., He, Z., Zhu, H., Hou, H. & Wang, L. (2011). Electrochemical and electrocatalytic properties of cobalt nanoparticles deposited on graphene modified glassy carbon electrode: Application to some amino acids detection. *Electrochim. Acta.*, *58*, 757–763.

[27] Yang, W., Ga, Z. o., Wang, J., Wang, B., Liu, Q. & Li, Z. (2012).Synthesis of reduced graphenenanosheet/urchin-like manganese dioxide composite and high performance as supercapacitor electrode. *Electrochim. Acta.*, *69*, 112–119.

[28] Zhou, Y., Yin, H., Meng, X., Xu, Z., Fu, Y. & Ai, S. (2012). Direct electrochemistry of sarcosine oxidase on graphene, chitosan and silver nanoparticles modified glassy carbon electrode and its biosensing for hydrogen peroxide. *Electrochim. Acta.*, *71*, 294–301.

[29] Ping, J., Wu, J., Wang, Y. & Ying, Y. (2012). Simultaneous determination of ascorbic acid, dopamine and uric acid using high-performance screen-printed graphene electrode. *Biosens. Bioelectron.*, *34*, 70–76.

[30] Sheng, Z. H., Zheng, X. Q., Xu, J. Y., Bao, W. J. & Wang, F.B. (2012). Electrochemical sensor based on nitrogen doped graphene: Simultaneous determination of ascorbic acid, dopamine and uric acid. *Biosens. Bioelectron.*, *34*, 125–131.

[31] Sun, C. L., Lee, H. H., Yang, J. M. & Wu, C.C.(2011). The simultaneous electrochemical detection of ascorbic acid, dopamine, and uric acid using graphene/size-selected Ptnanocomposites. *Biosens. Bioelectron.*, *26*, 3450–3455.

[32] Tian, X., Cheng, C., Yuan, H., Du, J., Xiao, D. & Xie, S.(2012). Simultaneous determination of L-ascorbic acid, dopamine and uric acid with gold nanoparticles-β-cyclodextrin-graphene- modified electrode by square wave voltammetry. *Talanta*, *93*, 79–85.

[33] Cong, H. L., Chen, J. & Cao, W. X. (2003). Covalently attached sandwich structure from colloidal particles and diazoresin. *J. Colloid Interface Sci.*, *263*, 665–668.

[34] Yu, B., Cong, H. L., Liu, H. W. & Wei, F. (2006). Fabrication and characterization of stable ultrathin film micropatterns containing DNA and photosensitive polymer diazoresin. *Anal. Bioanal. Chem.*, *384*, 385–390.

[35] Yang, Y. H. & Li, W. Z. (2011). Radial elasticity of single-walled carbon nanotube measured by atomic force microscopy. *Appl. Phy. Lett.*, *98*, 041901.

[36] Kroto, H. W., Heath, J. R. & O'Brien, S. C. (1985). C_{60}: Buckminster fullerene. *Nature.*, *318*, 162–164.

[37] Cho, J., Char, K., Hong, J. D. & Lee, K. B. (2001). Fabrication of highly ordered multilayer films using a spin self-assembly method. *Adv. Mater.*, *13*, 1076–1078.

[38] Grzelczak, M., Vermant, J., Furst, E. M. & Liz-Marzan, L. M. (2010). Directed self-assembly of nanoparticles. *ACS Nano.*, *4*, 3591–3605.

[39] Deng, R. H., Liu, S. Q., Li, J. Y., Liao, Y.G., Tao, J. & Zhu, J.T. (2012). Mesoporous block copolymer nanoparticles with tailored structures by hydrogen-bonding-assisted self-assembly.*A dv. Mater.*, *24*, 1889–1983.

[40] Pompeo, F. & Resasco, D. E.(2002). Water solubilization of single-walled carbon nanotubes by functionalization with glucosamine. *Nano Lett.*, *2*, 369–373.

[41] Yu, B., Cui, W., Cong, H. L., Jiao, M.M., Liu, P. & Yang, S. J. (2013). A novel diazoresin/polyethylene glycol covalent capillary coating for analysis of proteins by capillary electrophoresis. *RSC Adv.*, *3*, (2013) 20010–20015.

[42] Yu, B., Liu, X. M., Cong, H. L., Wang, Z. H. & Tang, J. G. (2013). Fabrication of stable ultrathin transparent conductive graphe nemicropatterns using layer by layer self-assembly. *Sci. Adv. Mater.*, *5*, 1533–1538.

In: New Developments in Dopamine Research ISBN: 978-1-63484-789-6
Editor: Glen Hopkins

Chapter 2

Modulation of the Dopamine Synthesis and Release in the Retina: Light, Melatonin and Clock Genes

Lucia de Fatima Sobral Sampaio*
Laboratory of Biochemistry of the Central Nervous System Development,
Biological Sciences Institute, Federal University of Para,
Belém, PA, Brazil

Abstract

There is a vast literature about the dopamine importance in the retinal physiology and pathophysiology. Additionally, the vertebrate retina is a good model to study neurological diseases caused by disturbs in dopamine neurochemistry, since this tissue contains a complete dopaminergic system. The enzyme limiting of the velocity in the dopamine synthesis is the tyrosine hydroxylase (TH).

In the retina, TH is located in a subpopulation of the interneurons known as amacrine cells and interplexiform cells. Dopamine levels present a diurnal circadian behavior for the reason that they are modulated by light, clock genes and melatonin. The dopamine synthesis and release are inhibited by the nocturnal pineal hormone melatonin through a mechanism still devoid of the investigation. Melatonin is mainly produced by photoreceptors and melatonin membrane receptors

* Corresponding author: Lucia de Fatima Sobral Sampaio. Address: Av. Augusto Corrêa, No.1. Belém. PA. Brasil. CEP:66075-110. E-mail: lsampaio@ufpa.br.

are located in amacrine cells from retinas of all vertebrates studied, including humans. These receptors signalize mainly by Gi protein, however the melatonin pathway used in the modulation of the dopamine release does not include the inhibition of the cAMP levels, at least in chick retina development. This chapter presents a discussion about the modulation of the dopamine synthesis and release in the retina by light, clock genes and melatonin.

Keywords: dopamine, tyrosine hydroxylase, clock genes, light, melatonin, retina

INTRODUCTION

The main fact about dopamine (4-(2-aminoethyl)-benzene-1-2-diol) is that it is the main neurotransmitter in photopic vision, in learning and in sensations of pleasure (Dopamine search in PubMed retrieved 143039 publications in December, 30, 2015). Biochemically, dopamine metabolism occurs mainly in the citosol of the dopaminergic neurons. It is a catecholamine synthetized from tyrosine in two main steps, initiating by the transformation of the tyrosine in L-DOPA (L-3, 4-di-hidroxy-phenylalanine) by the enzyme tyrosine hydroxylase (tyrosine 3-monooxygenase; EC 1.14.16.2; TH), which is the rate-limiting enzyme in the dopamine synthesis. Next, dopamine is produced by L-DOPA decarboxylation that takes place into the enzyme Aromatic L-amino acid decarboxylase (dopa decarboxylase; EC 4.1.1.28). Dopamine suffer prompt autoxidation generating reactive ortho-quinone, and, because this, it is under highly regulated synthesis, vesicular uptake and inactivation processes in the citosol of the dopaminergic neurons (reviewed in Sampaio, 2013).

Regarding dopamine neurochemistry, this transmitter has vesicular uptake, vesicular storage, synaptic release and reuptake by selective membrane transporters (reviewed in Cheng et al., 2006). The dopamine receptors are grouped in D_1 and D_2 classes in function of the type of the modulation on adenylate cyclase enzyme (AC, EC 4.6.1.1.) performed by them. The D1 class of the dopamine receptors contains the D1 and D5 receptors that stimulate the AC by activation of the $G_{s/olf}$ subfamily of the G proteins, while the D_2, D_3 and D_4 dopamine receptors inhibit the AC activity by coupling to $G_{i/o}$ subfamily of the G proteins (reviewed in Beaulieu & Gainetdinov, 2011; Zang et al., 2014). These receptors can also be found assembled in homodimers, heterodimers and tetramers (Karpa et al., 2000; Franco et al., 2000; Casadó et al., 2009; Przybyla & Watts, 2010; Herrick-Davis et al., 2013; Guitart et al., 2014; Jorg et al., 2014).

In the retinal physiology, dopamine is the main transmitter in photopic vision, including the non-image forming vision. It is also related to photoreceptor metabolism and modulation of the release of the neurotransmitter (reviewed in Nguyen-Legros & Hicks, 2000; Witkovsky, 2004). Selective antibodies against TH were used to localize dopaminergic neurons in the retina. These two types of cells are firstly a subpopulation of the rounded amacrine cells, sparsely distributed in the inner nuclear layer and secondly the interplexiform cells. The TH-positive amacrine cells distribution is evolutionarily preserved, suggesting a common function for dopamine in retinal physiology of the vertebrates (Savy et al., 1989; Versaux-Botteri et al., 1992; Witkovsky & Schutte, 1991; Vigh et al., 2000; Reis et al., 2007). The distribution of the enzyme dopa decarboxylase normally accompanies the distribution of the TH, but it was also achieved alone in photoreceptors of the mammalian (Nguyen-Legros et al., 1994) and avian retinas (da Silva et al., 2009). The released dopamine binds pre- and post-synaptic receptors. As it rapidly diffuses throughout the retina, the binding to post-synaptic dopamine receptors can occur far from dopaminergic cells (reviewed in Nguyen-Legros et al., 1999). The final of the dopaminergic synapse occurs by selective dopamine uptake done by transporters located in the synaptic terminal of the dopaminergic amacrine cells (Cheng et al., 2006) and by non-selective transporters localized in ganglion cells, in horizontal cells, in photoreceptors and in retinal pigment epithelial cells. Up to now, these non-selective transporters were not observed in the retina of the avian species, but they were in retinas of the mammalian species (Rajan et al., 2000). The presence of the non-selective membrane transporters located in cells far from the place of the dopamine release is in agreement with a signaling by volume transmission postulated for TH-amacrine cells (Bejelk et al., 1996). Therefore, in the eye, dopamine acts locally as a neurotransmitter or diffusely as a neurohormone.

The distribution of the dopamine receptors in retinal neural and non-neural cells offers morphological substrate for dopamine functions in the retina (reviewed in Nguyen-Legros & Hicks, 2000; Witkovsky, 2004). In gold fish retina, the D_1 receptor was localized in horizontal and amacrine cells, in interplexiform cells, in bipolar cells, in ganglion cells, in Müller cells and in both plexiform layers (Behrens & Wagner, 1995; Mora-Ferrer et al., 1999). In chick retina, D_2/D_3 receptors are in amacrine cells, in inner segments of the photoreceptors and in both outer and inner plexiform layers, while D_4 receptor is in photoreceptors (Rohrer & Stell, 1995). In mammalian retinas, D_1 receptor distribution includes amacrine cells, bipolar cells, ganglion cells and both outer and inner plexiform layers (Nguyen-Legros et al., 1997). The D_2 receptor was mainly localized in all TH-positive amacrine cells and throughout the inner plexiform layer, including processes of the non TH-positive amacrine cells, while the D_4 receptor was observed only in photoreceptor inner segments (Derouiche & Asan, 1999). The D_5 receptor distribution was in pigment epithelium, some types of amacrine and in ganglion cells (Versaux-Botteri et al., 1997; Nguyen-Legros et al., 1999). Up to now, it was not shown dopamine receptors forming homo or hetero dimers in the retina, but this possibility cannot be discarded.

Disturbs in the dopamine machinery during early stages of the eye development are related with the pathophysiology of the myopia (Nebbioso et al., 2014). Additionally, the presence of the complete dopaminergic system in the retina transforms this tissue in a model to study neurological disturbs in dopaminergic areas of the brain, such as Parkinson disease, which curses with abnormality in retinal dopaminergic system too (Archibald et al., 2011; Tian et al., 2011). Despite of the importance in vision physiology and pathophysiology, some points of the dopamine synthesis and release in the retina are still not completely clear. This chapter presents a discussion about the modulation of the dopamine synthesis and release by their main modulators light, melatonin and clock genes.

The Tyrosine Hydroxylase Enzyme (TH)

Because TH is the rate-limiting step in the synthesis of the catecholamine, which in the case of the retina is the dopamine, we found that the current achievements about the kinetics and modulation of this enzyme is the best background in a discussion about modulation of the dopamine synthesis and release by light melatonin and clock genes.

The TH is a member of a family of the enzymes that perform the hydroxylation in the aromatic rings of the amino acids. Each one of these enzymes has a homo tetramer structure, with each subunit presenting a multi-domain structure with an N-terminal regulatory domain (R), a C-terminal catalytic domain (C) and a coiled-coil domain at the carboxyl terminal. Indeed, the catalysis occurs by means of the non-heme ferrous iron atom. To transform the tyrosine in L-DOPA, TH uses diatomic oxygen and reduced biopterin (tetrahydrobiopterin, BH4) in a reaction on the iron atom, which is coordinated with two histidine residues and a glutamate residue in the active site (reviewed in Ledley et al., 1985; Roberts & Fitzpatrick, 2013).

The L-DOPA is transformed in dopamine by dopa decarboxylase. Therefore, the TH quantity and intrinsic activity indicate the amount of the dopamine that will be produced, and, then, can be released. This is important because the distances covered by dopamine diffusion to targets (dopamine receptors) far from the dopaminergic cells is dependent on the amount of the dopamine released (volume transmission) (Bejelk et al., 1996; reviewed in Tekin et al., 2014). As other catecholamines that present toxicity devoid to their capability of the autoxidation to catechol quinones, with parallel production of free radicals (reviewed in Sampaio, 2013), the dopamine has not a continuous constitutive rate of the synthesis. Henceforth, the dopamine levels are under a use-dependent replenishment (Kummer et al., 1996). In function of the potential toxicity, the excess of the cytosolic dopamine is inactivated through methylation (Catechol O-methyl transferase (COMT, EC 2.1.1.6) or oxidation (Monoamine oxidase (MAO, EC 1.4.3.4) (Hanna, 1965). Additionally, the non-uptacked excess of the L-dopa and dopamine in the cytosol suffers autoxidation, generating dopaquinone and dopamine quinone. Both ortho-quinones are the substrate of the cytosolic enzyme NRH: Quinone Oxidoreductase 2 (Ribosyl dihydronicotinamide dehydrogenase (quinone); QR2; EC 1.10.99.2). Thus, the product of the QR2 catalysis is either dopamine or L-DOPA recovered by double reduction (Sampaio et al., 2014; Cassagnes et al., 2015), in parallel, QR2 activity generates free radicals and toxic quinones. This potential toxicity has put QR2 as a target for inhibitors (Cassagnes et al., 2015; Sampaio et al., 2015).

The modulation of the TH activity can be classified in the short term or the medium-long term, which comprises modulators of the TH synthesis and expression.

The short term direct regulation of the TH activity includes negative feed-back, inhibitors, allosteric modulation and phosphorylation. Therefore, the TH activity can be inhibited either through binding of the catecholamine products or excess of the substrate. TH is under modulation by phosphorylation and protein-protein binding too. The catechol products bind the iron in the active site, inducing inhibition in the TH activity by covering the reduced biopterin binding site. Different of the negative feed-back, the TH positive modulation by phosphorylation occurs at R domain level, which phosphorylated induces reduction in the L-dopa and dopamine affinity at active site. Thus, the modulation by negative feed-back can be hampered by activation of the any signaling pathway that actives one or more of the following enzymes: cAMP-dependent Protein Kinase (PKA, EC 2.7.11.11), Ca^{2+}/Diacylglycerol-dependent Protein Kinase (PKC, EC 2.7.11.13), Ca^{2+}/Calmodulin-dependent Protein Kinase (CAMKII, EC 2.7.11.17), Extracellular Regulated Protein Kinase (EC 2.7.11.24) 1 and 2 (ERK1 and ERK2), and other kinases. The phosphorylation occurs at Ser 8, -19, -31 and -40. The Ser at position 8 is replaced by threonine in some species, including human, augmenting much more the TH resilience to negative feed-back (reviewed in Daubner et al., 2011; Tekin et al., 2014). The sites of the phosphorylation in the TH-R domain are also targets of the Serine/threonine protein phosphatase PP2A (EC 3.1.3.16). The dephosphorylation facilitates the inhibition of the TH activity by the catecholamine binding in the active site.

The TH activation via phosphorylation is modulates by interaction protein-protein. The binding of the 14-3-3 proteins enhances much more the resilience to negative-feedback produced by phosphorylation, not only at Ser-40, but also, and principally, at Ser-19. Another interesting protein-protein modulation occurs by the protein α-synuclein, which inhibits the PP2A, causing increased TH activity. To end with, the nitration of the TH at three tyrosine residues by nitric oxide (NO) and superoxide results in loss of enzymatic activity (reviewed in Daubner et al., 2011; Dickson & Briggs, 2013). Taken together, the short term modulation of the dopaminergic TH is in function of the trans-synaptic events in the retina.

The medium to long term regulation of the dopaminergic tyrosine hydroxylase occurs at transcriptional and post-transcriptional levels, the last including the modulation by miRNAs. The TH-gene has specie-, context- and development-dependent regulation. The specific starter of the dopaminergic TH-gene occurs by the appearing of the Nurr1 (Nuclear receptor related-1), an orphan nuclear receptor, which is expressed in the development by action of the isoleukin-1β, and that, mainly together with the transcription factor Pitx1/3 (Pituitary homeobox 1/3), it is responsible for the differentiation and maintenance of the dopaminergic neurons. It occurs by Nurr1 biding in the Nurr1 response binding element and Pitx1/3 bind sites that are located in the promoter, which is in a region upstream of the dopaminergic TH-gene. Nurr1 has an ERK1/ERK2 phosphorilation site that is related to activation of this nuclear receptor. Other transcription factors and silencers participate with Nurr1 of the differentiation and maintenance of the phenotype of the dopaminergic neurons, as recently reviewed. Whether Nurr1 activates the transcription of the dopaminergic TH-gene by binding directly or indirectly to promoter, it is dependent on the species used in the study. Dopaminergic TH-gene promoter also has binding sites for several other Nurr1 independent transcription factors (Kumer & Vrana, 1996; Lenartowski & Goc, 2011; reviewed in Tekin et al., 2014).

In vivo studies showed increase in TH mRNA levels, and, depending upon the duration of the stimulus, increase in protein levels, when rats were submitted to cold/immobilization stress or other stimulus that changes the physiological state of the animal, causing membrane depolarization. TH mRNA concentrations are also modulated by drug administration (glucocorticoids, nicotine, reserpine, dopamine antagonist, etc.). As was also shown to occur in the presence of the stressors, these drugs trigger pathways that activate the expression of the selective transcription factors. The TH-gene promoter region contains the following modulatory binding sites: GRE, glucocorticoid regulatory element that binds glucocorticoids; AP-1, the site of the transcription factor FOS/JUN immediate early protein binding site; CRE, cAMP-responsive element that binds CREB (cAMP-responsive element binding protein); HIF-1, oxygen regulated element; NFKb-like motif; AP-2 sites (2) and SP-1 site. The control of the TH-gene tissue specific expression is located in a dyad at EBOX region of the promoter that bind the proteins CDP2 and rlTF2 complexed. In addition, a heptamer sequence (HEPT) between the CRE and AP-1/E-BOX dyad sequences binds OCT-2, which is an inhibitor. Finally, we highlighted the importance of the presence of the second messengers Ca^{2+} and cAMP to expression of the dopaminergic TH-gene, because they trigger, respectively, the PKCAMII and PKA pathways that are the messengers linked to activation of the dopaminergic TH-gene transcription factors (reviewed in Kumer & Vrana, 1996; Lenartowski & Goc, 2011; Tekin et al., 2014). Thus, the medium- to long- term modulation of the TH levels can also be under trans-synaptic stimulus modulation.

In relation to TH turnover, the stability of the TH appears to depend of the prompt switch between the allosteric states TH-active, TH-less active and TH-inactive. This occurs because the TH-active has phosphoSer40, which leads to altered tertiary structure and, then, less stability. The same occurs in the presence of the ascorbate or BH4, while the inhibitors previously cited increase the TH stability by preventing phosphorilation. The phosphorylation at Ser 19 and 40 is the signal to ubiquitination in Rat TH and human TH. Subsequently, the TH-ubiquitin complex goes to degradation inside the proteasome (reviewed in Nakashima et al., 2013; Tekin et al., 2014). Therefore, the stability of the enzyme depends of the imbalance between the phosphorylation and the dephosphorylation of the critical amino acids, as was discussed before, in this chapter.

Modulation by Light of the Dopamine Synthesis and Release

In the retina, the light triggers electric signals in neural circuits related to both image forming vision (IFV) and non-image forming vision (NIFV). The IFV pathway is elicited by light stimulating opsins present in cones and rods photoreceptors (Field & Chichilnisky, 2007), while the NIFV is started by light simulating melanopsins present in a specific type of the ganglion cell named intrinsically photosensitive melanopsin-expressing retinal ganglion cells (mRGC) (Hattar et al., 2002; Zhao et al., 2014; Reifler et al., 2015). The NIFV is related to the photic entrainment of the circadian rhythm (Ruby et al., 2002), pupil size (Lucas et al., 2003) and sleep (Lupi et al., 2008). As a photic event, dopamine synthesis and release are generated by light sensitizing melanopsin and opsins (Cameron et al., 2009).

The main transmitter in the IFV is glutamate, which is released by photoreceptors in the scotopic vision and by bipolar cells in the photic vision. In brief, the light stops the glutamate release from photoreceptors and depolarizes bipolar cells. This occurs because the absence of the glutamate binding to mGluR6 (metabotropic glutamate receptor 6) results in membrane depolarization and glutamate release from bipolar cells (reviewed in Tian & Kammermeier, 2006). The glutamate released by bipolar cells can trigger phosphorylation cascades in dopaminergic amacrine cells, either directly by its proper glutamate metabotropic receptors or non-directly by activating ionotropic glutamate receptors that are capable to trigger the release of the other neurotransmitters. Thus, the increase in TH activity by light is a trans-synaptic event in the IFV, which curses by an excitatory glutamatergic increase in phosphorilation cascades in dopaminergic neurons.

Another trans-synaptic event mediated by light is the expression of the transcription factors that bind in the promoter region of the TH-gene, as previously described in this chapter. In mammalian retina, among the most studied cascade of the light expressed transcription factor is: Light → cFOS → FOS → AP1. As matter or fact, no FOS was observed at dark adapted retina in the ganglion cell layer and in the proximal border of INL, where dopaminergic, cholinergic and NOS- containing amacrine cells are found (McCormack & Burnside, 1993; Koistinaho & Sagar, 1996). Therefore, the light-increased TH activity can be accompanied of the light-induced increase in TH-mRNA levels. However, the full effectiveness of the TH production occurs only when the light stimulus is applied in phase with the circadian rhythm of the production of this enzyme (reviewed in Tekin et al., 2014). On the other hand, when the retina has prolonged exposition to light or dark, retinal clocks prompt the entrainiment of the circadian rhythmic synthesis and release of the dopamine in mammalian species (Rea, 1998; Ribelayga et al., 2004; Bobu et al., 2013).

Modulation of the Dopamine Synthesis and Release by Clock Genes

The retina functioning is under the circadian rhythm driven by local biological clocks that work doing temporal organization, even in the absence of the environmental light or dark signals. Therefore, the dopamine synthesis and release are fully dependent not only of the light, but they also are in function of the rhythmic expression of the retinal clock genes.

Different of the master clock (Suprachiasmatic nuclei of hypothalamus), the local retinal clocks are much more susceptible to be set by environmental luminance. The core of this intricate molecular machinery is formed mainly by the Period genes Per1 and Per2, Cryptochrome genes Cry1 and Cry2 and the transcription factors Clock and Bmal1. These transcription factors activate the production of the Per and Cry proteins that form a heterodimer, which returns to the nucleus inhibiting the Clock and Bmall binding to promoter. To this fundamental negative feedback looping is added a second loop, in which, the daily rhythm of the Bamal1 transcription is produced (reviewed in McMahon et al., 2014).

In retinas from mammalian species, the regulation of the clock machinery is much more intricate than in non-mammalian species. Additionally, a little expression of the clock genes in photoreceptors is observed in retinas from mammalian species, if compared with the quantity of the clock genes mRNA achieved in retinas from non-mammalian species. However, the clock genes mRNA and their proteins are present in all dopaminergic amacrine neurons from retinas of all species studied. Dopaminergic amacrine neurons also have the highest rate of the clock proteins, establishing these neurons as an important control place of the retinal circadian rhythmicity, through dopamine levels reaching to high values during the subjective day. The production and release of the dopamine are the signal of the light phase to other retinal rhythmic events. Further than TH rhythmicity, the expression of the D_4 dopamine receptor in photoreceptors also is under clock genes control (reviewed in McMahon et al., 2014; Jaeger et al., 2015; Sollars & Pickard, 2015). The activity of this dopamine receptor (Patel et al., 2003) inhibits the melatonin release, marking the final of the dark phase in the retinal circadian rhythm.

The complexity of the molecular machinery to control the circadian events in retinal physiology in mammalian species also includes layer-specific oscillators (Jaeger et al., 2015). Additionally, in mouse retinas with absence of the melanopsin, both the light-dependent expression of the retinal clocks Per1 and Per2 in photoreceptors and the positive modulation by light of the dopamine synthesis and release in amacrine cells are not shown to occur. These evidences are in agreement with the importance of the backward signaling pathways from mRGC to photoreceptors and from mRGC to amacrine cells to expression and control of the retinal clocks and dopamine levels (Dkhissi-Benyahya et al., 2013).

Melatonin Modulation of the Dopamine Synthesis and Release

In all vertebrates, melatonin is the pineal hormone that entrains the dark signal in the cell functioning. Melatonin takes place in almost all physiological events related to sleep and dark phase of the circadian rhythm. The normal embryonic and fetal development is dependent on the melatonin presence. Furthermore, this hormone is an anti-inflammatory agent. In the retinal physiology, melatonin is the principal transmitter in both photic rod dark adapted and non-photic events (Melatonin search in PubMed retrieved 20846 publications in December, 30, 2015).

In the retinal photoreceptors, melatonin synthesis is inhibited by both light and the activity of the D4 dopamine receptor (Cahill & Besharse, 1991; Tosine & Dirden, 2000). Regarding melatonin synthesis, the enzyme limiting of the velocity is the Arylalkilamine N-acetyltransferase (AANAT, EC 2.13.87). The increase in AANAT levels occurs by activation of the CRE and Clock-Bmal1 protein complex binding in specific promoter regions of the AANAT-gene (reviewed in Tosini & Fukuhara, 2003). Interestingly, the AC1-gene also has a specific region, where the Bmal1-Clock protein complex binds into. Therefore, the cAMP upsurge that stimulates CRE occurs by circadian positive modulation of the synthesis of the AC1 enzyme in photoreceptors (Fukuhara et al., 2004). On the other hand, the trans-synaptic events triggered by melatonin binding to melatonin membrane receptors and binding sites modulate the expression of the retinal clock genes (Hiragaki et al., 2014). Regarding dopamine synthesis and release, melatonin triggers increase in both glutamate (Faillace et al., 1996) and GABA levels, resulting in the inhibition of the dopamine synthesis and release in amacrine cells (Boatright et al., 1994).

Melatonin membrane receptors from non-mammalian (Mel1a, Mel1b and Mel1c) and mammalian (MT1, MT2 and GPR50) species were cloned. These receptors are not always located in the same type of the retinal cells, as had been reviewed (Wiechmann et al., 2013).

Melatonin receptors activity has as a result mainly the activation of the G_i protein, leading to inhibition of the cAMP levels. Furthermore, the MT1 (Mel1a) receptor is associated with the activation of the G_q protein, which activates the phospholipase C enzyme (PLC, EC 3.1.4.11), in a pathway that courses with the elevation of the Ca^{+2} and diacylglycerol (DAG) levels and activation of the PKC. These effects are enhanced when triggered by MT1/MT2 heteromers. Interestingly, the ERK pathway can also be activated by both Gi protein and PKC, downstream to melatonin receptors. Furthermore, the MT2 (Mel1b) receptor is related to inhibition of the soluble form of the Guanylate cyclase (sGC, EC 4.6.1.2), with consequent inhibition of the cGMP levels (reviewed in Tosini et al., 2014). Melatonin also inhibits the calcium binding protein calmodulin (de Almeida-Paula et al., 2005) and binds to retinoid-related orphan receptors (RORs) (Reviewed in Jetten, 2009).

Dopamine has rhythmic retinal levels inhibited by melatonin in all species studied (Nowak et al., 1992; Boatright et al., 1994; Behreus et al., 2000; Doyle et al., 2002). The inhibition of the dopamine release is an effect triggered by activation of the melatonin membrane receptors because it is blocked by the non-selective antagonist luzindole in *in vitro* (Dubocovich, 1983; Dubocovich, 1988) and *in situ* experiments (Ribelayga et al., 2004; Sampaio et al., 2014). The subtype of the melatonin receptor candidate to trigger the inhibition of the dopamine release is the MT1(Mel1a). This receptor is functional in mRGC (Pack et al., 2015) and in both dopaminergic and GABAergic amacrine cells from mammalian retinas (Fujieda et al., 2000), including retinas from macaque and human (Scher et al., 2003), while MT2 (Mel1b) is not present in dopaminergic amacrine cells (Wiechmann et al., 2004). Nevertheless, in these retinal neurons, the pathway, or pathways, used by MT1(Mel1a) to control dopamine levels is still not known. The more plausible possibility is melatonin modulating dopamine release and synthesis by different pathways. The pathway of the first effect should be a simple pre-synaptic event triggered by membrane receptor and, of the second, must be a more intricate pathway, including the control of the retinal clock genes machinery by melatonin.

Since MT1 (Mel1a) melatonin receptor co-localizes with TH in amacrine cells, the inhibition of the cAMP levels, leading to inactivation of the PKA can reduce the TH activity, which depends of the PKA phosphorylation. The same occurs by melatonin inhibition of the cAMP levels triggered by calmodulin (de Almeida-Paula et al., 2005). However, melatonin action on melatonin receptors and binding sites can increase other enzymes that activate the TH by phosphorylation (reviewed in this chapter), such as PKC (Zhao et al., 2010). Melatonin still activates the ERK pathway, which can translocate to the nucleus to trigger both TH synthesis (reviewed in this chapter) and rhythmicity in the levels of this enzyme.

At present, neither the mechanism underlying the modulation of the dopamine release nor the pathway used by melatonin in the inhibition of the dopamine synthesis was investigated in developing mammalian retinas. However, the melatonin inhibition on basal and stimulated cAMP levels in chick non-differentiated retinas were not blocked by luzindole (Sampaio, 2008), while this melatonin non-selective antagonist increased the endogenous levels of the dopamine in the same preparation (Sampaio et al., 2014). These achieves are in favor of the melatonin is inhibiting the dopamine release by a mechanism non-mediate by cAMP, at least in non-differentiated neural tissues.

Conclusion

In the retina, the dopamine synthesis and release are dependent on trans-synaptic events triggered by light. However, in constant light, the rhythmic levels of the dopamine are driven by clock genes through melatonin action on melatonin receptors. Despite of the unknowing on the pathway used, the control of the rhythmic synthesis of the dopamine takes part in the circadian events modulated by melatonin.

References

Archibald, N. K., Clarke, M. P., Mosimann, U. P. and Burn, D. J. (2011). Retinal thickness in Parkinson's disease. *Parkinsonism Relat. Disord.*, 17, 431-436.

Beaulieu, J. M. and Gainetdinov, R. R. (2011). The physiology, signaling, and pharmacology of dopamine receptors. *Pharmacol. Rev.*, 63, 182-217.

Bhrens, U. D. and Wagner, H. J. (1995). Localization of dopamine D1-receptors in vertebrate retinae. *Neurochem. Int.*, 27, 497-507.

Bjelke, B., Goldstein, M., Tinner, B., Andersson, C., Sesack, S.R., Steinbusch, H.W., Lew, J.Y., He, X., Watson, S., Tengroth, B. and Fuxe, K. (1996). Dopaminergic transmission in the rat retina: evidence for volume transmission. *J. Chem. Neuroanat.,* 12, 37-50.

Boatright, J.H, Rubim, N.M. and Iuvone, P.M. (1994). Regulation of endogenous dopamine release in amphibian retina by melatonin: the role of GABA. *Vis Neurosci.*, 11, 1013-1018.

Bobu, C., Sandu, C., Laurent, V., Felder-Schmittbuhl, M. P. and Hicks, D. (2013). Prolonged light exposure induces widespread phase shifting in the circadian clock and visual pigment gene expression of the Arvicanthis ansorgei retina. *Mol. Vis.*, 19, 1060-1073.

Cameron, M. A., Pozdeyev, N., Vugler, A. A., Cooper, H., Iuvone, P. M., Lucas, R. J. (2009). Light regulation of retinal dopamine that is independent of melanopsin phototransduction. *Eur. J. Neurosci.*, 29, 761-767.

Cahill, G.M. and Besharse, J.C. (1991). Resetting the circadian clock in cultured Xenopus eyecups: regulation of retinal melatonin rhythms by light and D2 dopamine receptors. *J. Neurosci.,* 11, 2959-2971.

Casadó, V., Ferrada, C., Bonaventura, J., Gracia, E., Mallol, J., Canela, E. I., Lluís, C., Cortés, A. and Franco R. (2009). Useful pharmacological parameters for G-protein-coupled receptor homodimers obtained from competition experiments. Agonist-antagonist binding modulation. *Biochem. Pharmacol.*, 78, 1456-1463.

Cassagnes, L. E., Perio, P., Ferry, G., Moulharat, N., Antoine, M., Gayon, R., Boutin, J. A., Nepveu, F. and Reybier, K. (2015). In cellulo monitoring of quinone reductase activity and reactive oxygen species production during the redox cycling of 1,2 and 1,4 quinones. *Free Radic. Biol. Med.*, 89, 126-134.

Chaurasia, S.S., Haque, R., Pozdeyev, N., Jackson, C.R. and Iuvone, P.M. (2006). Temporal coupling of cyclic AMP and Ca/calmodulin-stimulated adenylyl cyclase to the circadian clock in chick retinal photoreceptor cells. *J. Neurochem.,* 99, 1142-1150.

Cheng, Z., Zhong, Y. M. and Yang, X. L. (2006). Expression of the dopamine transporter in rat and bullfrog retinas. *Neuroreport.*, 17, 773-777.

da Silva, R. T., Hokoç, J. N., de Mello, F. G. and Gardino, P. F. (2009). Differential immunodetection of L-DOPA decarboxylase and tyrosine hydroxylase in the vertebrate retina. *Int. J. Dev. Neurosci.*, 27, 469-476.

de Almeida-Paula, L.D., Costa-Lotufo, L.V., Silva Ferreira, Z., Monteiro, A.E., Isoldi, M.C., Godinho, R.O. and Markus, R.P. (2005). Melatonin modulates rat myotube-acetylcholine receptors by inhibiting calmodulin. *Eur. J. Pharmacol.*, 525, 24-31.

Dubner, S. C., Le, T. and Wang, S. (2011). Tyrosine hydroxylase and regulation of dopamine synthesis. *Arch. Biochem. Biophys.*, 508, 1-12.

Derouiche, A. and Asan, E. (1999). The dopamine D2 receptor subfamily in rat retina: ultrastructural immunogold and in situ hybridization studies. *Eur. J. Neurosci.*, 11, 1391-1402.

Dickson, P. W. and Briggs, G. D. (2013). Tyrosine hydroxylase: regulation by feedback inhibition and phosphorylation. *Adv. Pharmacol.*, 68, 13-21.

Dkhissi-Benyahya, O., Coutanson, C., Knoblauch, K., Lahouaoui, H., Leviel, V., Rey, C., Bennis, M. and Cooper, H. M. (2013). The absence of melanopsin alters retinal clock function and dopamine regulation by light. *Cell Mol. Life Sci.*, 70, 3435-3447.

Dorenbos, R., Contini, M., Hirasawa, H., Gustincich, S. and Raviola, E. (2007). Expression of circadian clock genes in retinal dopaminergic cells. *Vis. Neurosci.*, 24, 573-580.

Doyle, S.E., Grace, M.S., McIvor, W. and Menaker, M. (2002). Circadian rhythms of dopamine in mouse retina: the role of melatonin. *Vis. Neurosci.*, 19, 593-601.

Dubocovich, M.L. (1983). Melatonin is a potent modulator of dopamine release in the retina. *Nature*, 306, 782-784.

Dubocovich, M.L. (1988). Luzindole (N-0774): a novel melatonin receptor antagonist. *J. Pharmacol. Exp. Ther.*, 246, 902-910.

Faillace, M.P., Sarmiento, M.I. and Rosenstein, R.E. (1996). Melatonin effect on [3H] glutamate uptake and release in the golden hamster retina. *J. Neurochem.*, 67, 623-628.

Field, G. D. and Chichilnisky, E. J. (2007). Information processing in the primate retina: circuitry and coding. *Annu. Rev. Neurosci.*, 30, 1-30.

Franco, R., Ferré, S., Agnati, L., Torvinen, M., Ginés, S., Hillion, J., Casadó, V., Lledó, P., Zoli, M., Lluis, C. and Fuxe, K. (2000). Evidence for adenosine/dopamine receptor interactions: indications for heteromerization. *Neuropsychopharmacology*, 23, 50-59.

Fujieda, H., Scher, J., Hamadanizadeh, S.A., Wankiewicz, E., Pang, S.F. and Brown, G.M. (2000). Dopaminergic and GABAergic amacrine cells are direct targets of melatonin: immunocytochemical study of mt1 melatonin receptor in guinea pig retina. *Vis Neurosci.*, 17, 63-70.

Fukuhara, C., Liu, C., Ivanova, T.N., Chan, G.C., Storm, D.R., Iuvone, P.M. and Tosini G. (2004). Gating of the cAMP signaling cascade and melatonin synthesis by the circadian clock in mammalian retina. *J Neurosci.*, 24, 1803-1811.

Gitart, X., Navarro, G., Moreno, E., Yano, H., Cai, N. S., Sánchez-Soto, M., Kumar-Barodia, S., Naidu, Y.T., Mallol, J., Cortés, A., Lluís, C., Canela, E. I., Casadó, V., McCormick, P. J. and Ferré, S. (2014). Functional selectivity of allosteric interactions within G protein-coupled receptor oligomers: the dopamine D1-D3 receptor heterotetramer. *Mol Pharmacol.*, 86, 417-29.

Hanna, C. (1965). Metabolism of catecholamines. *Invest Ophthalmol*, 4, 1095-1104.

Hattar, S. Liao, H. W., Takao, M., Berson, D. M. and Yau, K. W. (2002). Melanopsin-containing retinal ganglion cells: architecture, projections, and intrinsic photosensitivity. *Science*, 295, 1065-1070.

Herick-Davis, K., Grinde, E., Cowan, A. and Mazurkiewicz, J. E. (2013). Fluorescence correlation spectroscopy analysis of serotonin, adrenergic, muscarinic, and dopamine receptor dimerization: the oligomer number puzzle. *Mol. Pharmacol.*, 84, 630-642.

Hiragaki, S., Baba, K., Coulson, E., Kunst, S., Spessert, R. and Tosini, G. (2014). Melatonin signaling modulates clock genes expression in the mouse retina. *PLoS One*. Sep. 9;9(9):e106819.

Icard-Liepkalns, C., Berrard, S., Faucon Biguet, N., Lebourdelles, B., Ravassard, P., Robert, J. J. and Mallet, J. (1993). Tyrosine hydroxylase regulation in neurotransmission and neuroplasticity. *J. Physiol.*, 87, 153-157.

Iuvone, P. M. and Neff, N. H. Dopamine neurons of the retina: a simple method system for studying synaptic regulatory mechanisms. *Essays Neurochem. Neuropharmacol.*, 5, 75-94.

Iuvone, P. M., Galli, C. L., Garrison-Gund, C. K. and Neff, N. H. (1978). Light stimulates tyrosine hydroxylase activity and dopamine synthesis in retinal amacrine neurons. *Science*, 202, 901-902.

Jager, C., Sandu, C., Malan, A., Mellac, K., Hicks, D. and Felder-Schmittbuhl, M. P. (2015) Circadian organization of the rodent retina involves strongly coupled, layer-specific oscillators. *FASEB J.*, 29, 1493-1504.

Jetten, A.M. (2009). Retinoid-related orphan receptors (RORs): critical roles in development, immunity, circadian rhythm, and cellular metabolism. *Nucl. Recept. Signal.*, 7:e003.

Jorg, M., Scammells, P. J. and Capuano, B. (2014). The dopamine D2 and adenosine A2A receptors: past, present and future trends for the treatment of Parkinson's disease. *Curr. Med. Chem.*, 21, 3188-31210.

Karpa, K. D., Lin, R., Kabbani, N. and Levenson, R. (2000). The dopamine D3 receptor interacts with itself and the truncated D3 splice variant d3nf: D3-D3nf interaction causes mislocalization of D3 receptors. *Mol. Pharmacol.*, 58, 677-683.

Koistinaho, J. and Sagar, S. M. (1995). Light-induced c-fos expression in amacrine cells in the rabbit retina. *Brain Res. Mol. Brain Res.*, 29, 53-63.

Kumer, S. C. and Vrana, K. E. (1996). Intricate regulation of tyrosine hydroxylase activity and gene expression. *J Neurochem.* 67, 443-462.

Kunst, S., Wolloscheck, T., Kelleher, D. K., Wolfrum, U., Sargsyan, S. A., Iuvone, P. M., Baba, K., Tosini, G. and Spessert, R. (2015). Pgc-1α and Nr4a1 Are Target Genes of Circadian Melatonin and Dopamine Release in Murine Retina. *Invest. Ophthalmol. Vis. Sci.*, 56, 6084-6094.

Ledley, F.D., DiLella, A.G., Kwok, S.M.C. and Woo, S.L.C. (1985). Homology between phenylalanine and tyrosine hydroxylases reveals common structural and functional domains. *Biochemistry*, 24, 3389-3394.

Lenartowski, R. and Goc, A. (2011). Epigenetic, transcriptional and posttranscriptional regulation of the tyrosine hydroxylase gene. *Int. J. Dev. Neurosci.*, 29, 873-883.

Lucas, R. J., Hattar, S., Takao, M., Berson, D. M., Foster, R. G. and Yau, K. W. (2003) Diminished pupillary light reflex at high irradiances in melanopsin-knockout mice. *Science*, 299, 245-247.

Lupi, D., Oster, H., Thompson, S. and Foster, R. G. (2008). The acute light-induction of sleep is mediated by OPN4-based photoreception. *Nat. Neurosci.*, 11, 1068-1073.

Maggio, R., Aloisi, G., Silvano, E., Rossi, M. and Millan, M. J. (2009). Heterodimerization of dopamine receptors: new insights into functional and therapeutic significance. *Parkinsonism Relat. Disord.*, 15, 2-7.

McCormack, C. A. and Burnside, B. (1993). Light and circadian modulation of teleost retinal tyrosine hydroxylase activity. *Invest. Ophthalmol. Vis. Sci.*, 34, 1853-1860.

McMahon, D.G., Iuvone, P.M. and Tosini, G. (2014). Circadian organization of the mammalian retina: from gene regulation to physiology and diseases. *Prog. Retin Eye Res.*, 39, 58-76.

Mora-Ferrer, C., Yazulla, S., Studholme, K. M. and Haak-Frendscho, M. (1999). Dopamine D1-receptor immunolocalization in goldfish retina. *J. Comp. Neurol.*, 411, 705-714.

Nakashima, A., Kaneko, Y.S., Kodani, Y., Mori, K., Nagasaki, H., Nagatsu, T. and Ota, A. (2013). Intracellular stability of tyrosine hydroxylase: phosphorylation and proteasomal digestion of the enzyme. *Adv. Pharmacol.*, 68, 3-11.

Nebbioso, M., Plateroti, A. M., Pucci, B. and Pescosolido, N. (2014). Role of the dopaminergic system in the development of myopia in children and adolescents. *J. Child Neurol.*, 29, 1739-1746.

Nguyen-Legros, J., Krieger, M. and Simon, A. (1994). Immunohistochemical localization of L-dopa and aromatic L-amino acid-decarboxylase in the rat retina. *Invest. Ophthalmol. Vis. Sci.*, 35, 2906-2915.

Nguyen-Legros, J., Simon, A., Caillé, I. and Bloch, B. (1997). Immunocytochemical localization of dopamine D1 receptors in the retina of mammals. *Vis. Neurosci.*, 14, 545-551.

Nguyen-Legros, J., Versaux-Botteri, C. and Vernier, P. (1999). Dopamine receptor localization in the mammalian retina. *Mol. Neurobiol.*, 19, 181-204.

Nguyen-Legros, J. and Hicks D. (2000). Renewal of photoreceptor outer segments and their phagocytosis by the retinal pigment epithelium. *Int. Rev. Cytol.*, 196, 245-313.

Nowak, J.Z., Kazula, A. and Gołembiowska, K. (1992). Melatonin increases serotonin N-acetyltransferase activity and decreases dopamine synthesis in light-exposed chick retina: *in vivo* evidence supporting melatonin-dopamine interaction in retina. *J. Neurochem.*, 59, 1499-14505.

Pack, W., Hill, D.D. and Wong, K.Y. (2015). Melatonin modulates M4-type ganglion-cell photoreceptors. *Neuroscience*, 303, 178-188.

Patel, S., Chapman, K.L., Marston, D., Hutson, P.H. and Ragan C.I. (2003). Pharmacological and functional characterisation of dopamine D4 receptors in the rat retina. *Neuropharmacology*, 44, 1038-1046.

Przybyla, J. A. and Watts, V. J. (2010). Ligand-induced regulation and localization of cannabinoid CB1 and dopamine D2L receptor heterodimers. *J. Pharmacol. Exp. Ther.*, 332, 710-719.

Rajan, P. D., Kekuda, R., Chancy, C. D., Huang, W., Ganapathy, V. and Smith, S. B. (2000). Expression of the extraneuronal monoamine transporter in RPE and neural retina. *Curr. Eye Res.*, 20, 195-204.

Rea, M. A. (1998). Photic entrainment of circadian rhythms in rodents. *Chronobiol. Int.*, 15, 395-423.

Reifler, A. N., Chervenak, A. P., Dolikian, M. E., Benenati, B. A., Meyers, B. S., Demertzis, Z. D., Lynch, A. M., Li, B. Y., Wachter, R. D., Abufarha, F. S., Dulka, E. A., Pack, W., Zhao, X. and Wong, K.Y. (2015). The rat retina has five types of ganglion-cell photoreceptors. *Exp. Eye Res.*, 130, 17-28.

Reis, R. A., Ventura, A. L., Kubrusly, R. C., de Mello, M. C. and de Mello, F. G. (2007). Dopaminergic signaling in the developing retina. *Brain Res. Rev.*, 54, 181-188.

Rielayga, C., Wang, Y. and Mangel, S. C. (2004). A circadian clock in the fish retina regulates dopamine release via activation of melatonin receptors. *J. Physiol.* 554, 467-482.

Roberts, K. M., and Fitzpatrick, P. F. (2013). Mechanisms of Tryptophan and Tyrosine Hydroxylase. *IUBMB Life*, 65, 350-357.

Rohrer, B. and Stell, W. K. (1995). Localization of putative dopamine D2-like receptors in the chick retina, using in situ hybridization and immunocytochemistry. *Brain Res.*, 695, 110-116.

Ruby, N. F., Brennan, T. J., Xie, X., Cao, V., Franken, P., Heller, H. C. and O'Hara, B. F. (2002). Role of melanopsin in circadian responses to light. *Science*, 298, 2211-2213.

Sampaio, Lde F. (2008). Melatonin inhibitory effect on cAMP accumulation in the chick retina development. *Int. J. Dev. Neurosci.*, 26, 277-282.

Sampaio, L.F.S. (2013). Catecholquinones as Substrates of the NRH: Quinone Oxidoreductase 2 in the Brain and Retina. In: S. C. Johnson, E.R. Price (Eds.). *Quinones: Occurrence, Medicinal Uses and Physiological Importance* (1, pp. 141-156). New York, NY: NOVA Publishers.

Sampaio, Lde F., Mesquita, F.P., de Sousa, P.R., Silva, J.L. and Alves, C.N. (2014). The melatonin analog 5-MCA-NAT increases endogenous dopamine levels by binding NRH: quinone reductase enzyme in the developing chick retina. *Int. J. Dev. Neurosci.*, 38, 119-126.

Sampaio, Lde F., Mesquita, F.P., de Sousa, P.R.M., Silva, J.L. and Alves, C.N. (2015). NRH: Quinone reductase activity results in the accumulation of endogenous dopamine in the retina. *Neurotransmitter* 2:e505.

Savy, C., Yelnik, J., Martin-Martinelli, E., Karpouzas, I. and Nguyen-Legros, J. (1989). Distribution and spatial geometry of dopamine interplexiform cells in the rat retina: I. Developing retina. *J Comp Neurol.*, 289, 99-110.

Scher, J., Wankiewicz, E., Brown, G.M. and Fujieda, H. (2003). AII amacrine cells express the MT1 melatonin receptor in human and macaque retina. *Exp. Eye Res.*, 77, 375-782.

Sollars, P. J. and Pickard, G. E. (2015). The Neurobiology of Circadian Rhythms. *Psychiatr. Clin. North Am.* 38, 645-665.

Tekin, I., Roskoski, R. Jr., Carkaci-Salli, N. and Vrana, K. E. (2014). Complex molecular regulation of tyrosine hydroxylase. *J. Neural Transm.*, 121, 1451-1481.

Tian, L. and Kammermeier, P. J. (2006). G protein coupling profile of mGluR6 and expression of G alpha proteins in retinal ON bipolar cells. *Vis. Neurosci.*, 23, 909-916.

Tian, T., Zhu, X. H. and Liu, Y. H. (2011). Potential role of retina as a biomarker for progression of Parkinson's disease. *Int. J. Ophthalmol.*, 4, 433-438.

Tosini, G. and Dirden, J.C. (2000). Dopamine inhibits melatonin release in the mammalian retina: *in vitro* evidence. *Neurosci. Lett.*, 286, 119-122.

Tosini, G. and Fukuhara, C. (2003). Photic and circadian regulation of retinal melatonin in mammals. *J. Neuroendocrinol.*, 15, 364-369.

Tosini, G., Owino, S., Guillaume, J.L. and Jockers, R. (2014). Understanding melatonin receptor pharmacology: latest insights from mouse models, and their relevance to human disease. *Bioessays*, 36, 778-787.

Versaux-Botteri, C., Verney, C., Zecevic, N. and Nguyen-Legros, J. (1992). Early appearance of tyrosine hydroxylase immunoreactivity in the retina of human embryos. *Brain Res. Dev. Brain Res.* 23, 69, 283-287.

Versaux-Botteri, C., Gibert, J. M., Nguyen-Legros, J. and Vernier P. (1997). Molecular identification of a dopamine D1b receptor in bovine retinal pigment epithelium. *Neurosci. Lett.*, 237, 9-12.

Vígh, J., Bánvölgyi, T. and Wilhelm, M. (2000). Amacrine cells of the anuran retina: morphology, chemical neuroanatomy, and physiology. *Microsc. Res. Tech.*, 50, 373-383.

Wiechmann, A.F., Udin, S.B. and Summers Rada, J.A. (2004). Localization of Mel1b melatonin receptor-like immunoreactivity in ocular tissues of Xenopus laevis. *Exp. Eye Res.*, 79, 585-594.

Wiechmann, A.F. and Sherry, D.M. (2013). Role of melatonin and its receptors in the vertebrate retina. *Int. Rev. Cell. Mol. Biol.*, 300, 211-242.

Witkovsky, P. and Schütte, M. (1991). The organization of dopaminergic neurons in vertebrate retinas. *Vis Neurosci.*, 7, 113-124.

Witkovsky, P. (2004) Dopamine and retinal function. *Doc. Ophthalmol.*, 108, 17-40.

Zhang, D-Q, Zhou, T-R and McMahon, D.G. (2007). Functional heterogeneity of retinal dopaminergic neurons underlying their multiple roles in vision. *J. Neurosci.* 27, 692-699.

Zhao, W.J., Zhang, M., Miao, Y., Yang, X.L. and Wang, Z. (2010). Melatonin potentiates glycine currents through a PLC/PKC signalling pathway in rat retinal ganglion cells. *J. Physiol.*, 588, 2605-2619.

Zhao, X., Stafford, B.K., Godin, A.L., King, W.M. and Wong, K.Y. (2014). Photoresponse diversity among the five types of intrinsically photosensitive retinal ganglion cells. *J. Physiol.*, 592, 1619-1636.

BIOGRAPHICAL SKETCH

***Name*: Lucia de Fatima S. Sampaio**

Affiliation: Federal University of Pará. Biological Sciences Institute.

Education: PhD in Biological Science (Physiology) at São Paulo State University, SP, Brazil.

Address: Av Augusto Corrêa, No. 1. Belém, PA. CEP: 66075-110.

Research and Professional Experience:

Biochemistry Associated Professor. Research Projects in Neurodevelopment focusing Biochemistry and Molecular Pharmacology.

Professional Appointments: Hard of the Group "Biochemistry of the Neurodevelopment," Classes, Lectures, Management of the Research Projects.

***Honors*:**

2013 Best Poster Award, FASEB Science Research Conference. Melatonin Biology Actions and Therapeutics.

***Publications Last Three Years*:**

Sampaio, Lde F., Mesquita, F.P., de Sousa, P.R.M., Silva, J.L., Alves, C.N., 2014. The melatonin analog 5-MCA-NAT increases endogenous dopamine levels by binding NRH: quinone reductase enzyme in the developing chick retina. *Int. J. Dev. Neurosci.* 38, 119-126.

Silva, R.N., Sampaio, L.F.S., 2014. Immunoreactivity of Mel1a-like melatonin receptor and NRH: Quinone reductase enzyme (QR2) in testudine whole embryo and in developing whole retinas. *Trends Dev. Biol.* 8, 39-46.

Sampaio, Lde F., Mesquita, F.P., de Sousa, P.R.M., Silva, J.L., Alves, C.N., 2015. NRH: Quinone reductase activity results in the accumulation of endogenous dopamine in the retina. *Neurotransmitter* 2:e505.

In: New Developments in Dopamine Research ISBN: 978-1-63484-789-6
Editor: Glen Hopkins

Chapter 3

DOPAMINE, ERECTILE FUNCTION AND SEXUAL BEHAVIOR: LAST DISCOVERIES AND POSSIBLE ADVANCES

Fabrizio Sanna*[*], *Maria Rosaria Melis* and *Antonio Argiolas
Department of Biomedical Sciences,
Section of Neuroscience and Clinical Pharmacology,
University of Cagliari, Cagliari, Italy

ABSTRACT

Among neurotransmitters involved in the control of erectile function and sexual behavior, dopamine is one of the most studied. Since the first pioneering studies done in the nineteen sixties, which revealed the facilitatory role of this neurotransmitter in sexual behavior, today it is well accepted that dopamine is deeply involved in both the anticipatory (appetitive and rewarding) and consummatory (penile erection and ejaculation) phases of sexual behavior. Dopamine influences sexual behavior by acting at the level of several brain areas (i.e., medial preoptic area, paraventricular nucleus of the hypothalamus and ventral tegmental area that contains the cell bodies of mesolimbic dopaminergic neurons projecting to the nucleus accumbens). The facilitation of sexual function

[*] Corresponding Author at: Department of Biomedical Sciences, Section of Neuroscience and Clinical, Pharmacology, University of Cagliari, Italy, Email: fabrizio.sanna@unica.it.

by dopamine is mediated mainly by the stimulation of receptors of the D_2 family (D_2, D_3 and D_4), with only a minor role for those of the D_1 family (D_1 and D_5). In spite of the large amount of preclinical studies showing a facilitatory role of D_2-like receptors in sexual behavior, scarce success was obtained with classic D_2-like agonists (mainly apomorphine), especially when compared to that obtained with locally acting phosphodiesterase type V inhibitors, in the treatment of erectile dysfunction in humans. The discovery of selective D_4 receptor agonists able to induce penile erection with potency similar to that of classic mixed D_2 agonists in male rats has reopened the research aimed at the identification of dopamine agonists useful for the treatment of erectile dysfunction in humans. This review summarizes the most recent findings on the role of central D_2, D_3 and D_4 receptors on erectile function and sexual behavior. These studies suggest that D_4 receptors may represent a valuable therapeutic target for the therapy of erectile dysfunction.

Keywords: dopamine, dopamine receptor subtypes, erectile function, sexual behavior

INTRODUCTION

Sexual behavior plays a main role in reproduction of all living animals, from insects to mammals, including humans. In mammals, it is organized in two main phases, anticipatory and consummatory, and several quantifiable parameters have been identified in each phase and in both males and females. These studies were done mainly in rats because of their availability, the well characterized sequence of copulatory behavior and its parameters in the male (see [1-5]), and of proceptive and receptive (lordotic) behavior in the female (see [6, 7]), although data on some other animal species are also available (see [8]). Penile erection, seminal emission and ejaculation characterize the consummatory phase of the male sexual response, while vaginal lubrication, clitoris erection and orgasm are typical of the female sexual response. These consummatory responses are preceded by an anticipatory, mainly appetitive phase, which includes motivation towards and searching of an adequate partner for copulation (see [3, 4]). Briefly, when sexual (visual, auditory, olfactory, tactile and in humans even imaginative) stimuli reach the central nervous system, neural pathways are activated which convey sexual information from the higher brain centers through the spinal cord and the autonomous nervous system to the genital apparatus to induce penile erection in males and vaginal lubrication/clitoris erection in females in order to make sexual intercourse, which will culminate with orgasm, feasible (see [4-16] and references therein).

It is well known that numerous neurotransmitters and neuropeptides are involved at central and peripheral level in the control of both phases of sexual behavior. Among neurotransmitters, the best known are dopamine, serotonin, glutamic acid, gamma-amminobutirric acid (GABA), and nitric oxide (see [12-14, 17-20]). They influence sexual behavior by acting in different brain areas, from the hypothalamus and its nuclei [e.g., lateral hypothalamus, paraventricular nucleus (PVN), ventromedial nucleus, arcuate nucleus], to the medial preoptic area (MPOA) and other brain areas, which include the ventral tegmental area (VTA), the nucleus accumbens (NAc), the prefrontal cortex, the hippocampus, the amygdala, the medulla oblongata and the spinal cord. In these brain areas neurotransmitters often interact in a concerted manner with neuropeptides, such as oxytocin, adrenocorticotropin (ACTH), α-melanocyte stimulating hormone (α-MSH) and opioid peptides (see [19-25]) in the control of several aspects of sexual behavior, from sexual performance to sexual motivation and arousal or both (see [17, 20, 25-29]).

Dopamine is certainly one of the neurotransmitters that play a key role in sexual behavior. Since the first pioneering studies done in the 1960s, which revealed the classic dichotomy dopamine-serotonin, with dopamine facilitating and serotonin inhibiting sexual behavior, respectively (see [20, 29]), numerous studies have shown that dopamine is deeply involved in both the anticipatory (appetitive and rewarding) and consummatory (penile erection and ejaculation) aspects of sexual behavior by acting at the level of different brain areas, mainly hypothalamic and limbic areas, as the PVN, the MPOA, the VTA and the NAc (e.g., the mesolimbic dopaminergic system, with dopaminergic neurons originating in the VTA and projecting to the NAc). The stimulation or the blockade of dopamine neurotransmission in these brain areas, for instance with drugs that selectively stimulate or block dopamine receptors, mainly of the D2 family, usually leads to a facilitation or to an inhibition, respectively, of various (anticipatory or consummatory) aspects of sexual behavior (i.e., sexual motivation, penile erection, copulation) (see [20, 30-33]) (Figure 1).

This lead to support the idea that dopamine has a facilitatory role on both the anticipatory and consummatory phases of sexual behavior, although some criticism on this idea has been raised (see [34]).

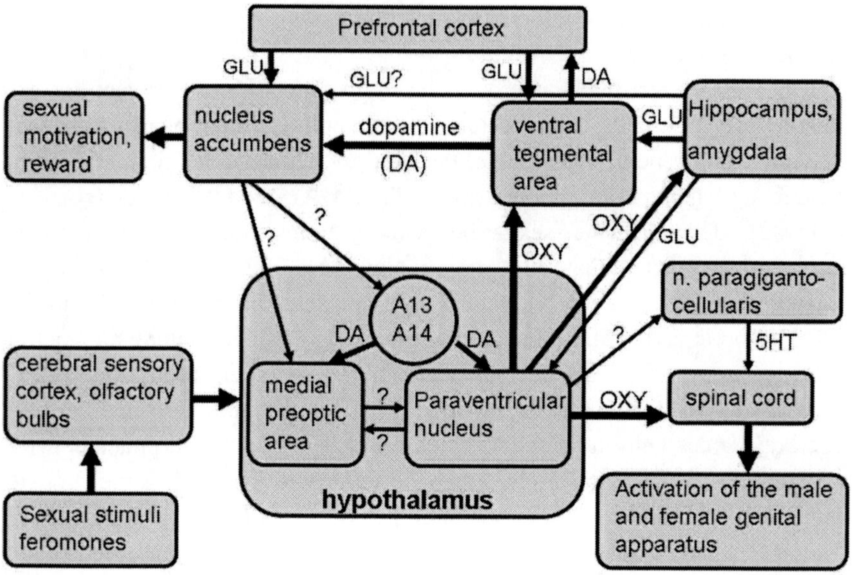

Figure 1. Schematic representation of a hypothetical neural circuitry involving dopamine, oxytocin and glutamic acid influencing sexual motivation, rewarding and sexual performance, as suggested by the results reviewed in this chapter and previous reports. Briefly, oxytocinergic neurons originating in the paraventricular nucleus and projecting to the spinal cord when activated for instance by dopamine and glutamic acid (but also by other neurotransmitters and/or neuropeptides), facilitate penile erection and sexual performance by activating oxytocinergic neurons projecting to the spinal cord. Dopamine and glutamic acid (but also other neurotransmitters and neuropeptides) in the paraventricular nucleus also activate oxytocinergic neurons projecting to the ventral tegmental area, thereby activating mesolimbic dopaminergic neurons projecting to the nucleus accumbens and the medial prefrontal cortex modulating sexual motivation and reward. Dopamine released in the nucleus accumbens and in the medial prefrontal cortex activates in turn still unknown neural pathways, which increase the activity of incerto-hypothalamic dopaminergic neurons (originating in the A13-A14 groups of Dahlstrom and Fuxe) impinging among others on oxytocinergic neurons, including those that project to the spinal cord, leading to penile erection. This circuitry may be also activated by oxytocin injected not only into the caudal ventral tegmental area, but also in the ventral subiculum of the hippocampus and in the amygdala, which also receive an oxytocinergic innervation from the paraventricular nucleus, possibly through direct or indirect glutamatergic efferents to the ventral tegmental area, leading to the modulation of both sexual motivation and penile erection. Finally, the above circuitry may be also activated by sexual stimuli and pheromones, since extracellular dopamine and glutamic acid increase in the paraventricular nucleus, and in the medial preoptic area as well, during pheromone–mediated noncontact erections and copulation (for appropriate references see the References list).

In line with such facilitatory role of dopamine in sexual behavior, the classical mixed dopamine receptor agonist apomorphine, well known for its ability to induce penile erection not only in laboratory animals, but also in humans, and to facilitate male copulatory behavior in laboratory animals, was made commercially available for the therapy of erectile dysfunction. However, the success of this preparation was scarce, especially when compared to that of orally and locally active phosphodiesterase type V inhibitors, possibly due to unwanted side effects of this and other dopamine agonists, such as nausea and vomiting, secondary to the stimulation of dopamine receptors located in the chemo-trigger zone outside the blood brain barrier (see [15] and references therein).

Table 1. Classification of dopamine receptors and their role in penile erection and copulatory behavior

Dopamine receptor family	Receptor subtypes	Transduction mechanisms	Role in penile erection	Role in copulatory behavior
D1	D_1	Increased activity of adenylate cyclase-cAMP signaling pathway, Increased PIP_2 turnover, Increased Ca^{2+} mobilization	None	None
	D_5		Not Available	Not Available
D2	D_{2s} - D_{2l}	Decreased activity of adenylate cyclase-cAMP signaling pathway, Increased K^+ channel activation, Increased voltage-gated Ca^{2+}channel activation	Facilitatory	Facilitatory
	D_3		None (but see [45])	Not Available
	D_4		Facilitatory (but see [45, 46])	Facilitatory

Appropriate references are quoted in the text.

The characterization of several dopamine receptors belonging to the D1 (D_1 and D_5) and D2 (D_2, D_3 and D_4) receptor families, has led in recent years to the synthesis of molecules that act selectively as agonists or antagonists of these dopamine receptor subtypes (Table 1). This has reopened the research aimed at the defining the exact role of the different dopamine receptor subtypes, mainly of the D2 family (D_2, D_3 and D_4), in the different aspects of sexual behavior, from sexual motivation to penile erection and copulatory behavior. During one of these studies, ABT-724, a selective D_4 receptor agonist, was found able to induce penile erection in male rats, with potency comparable to that of apomorphine, leading to suggest that the facilitatory effect of dopamine receptors of the D2 type was mainly due to the stimulation of D_4 receptors [35]. This discovery was soon followed by the identification of other selective D_4 receptor agonists able to induce penile erection in male rats [36-44] (Table 2), although some conflicting results have appeared in the literature on this point [45, 46].

The aim of this work is to review the most recent studies on the role of these recently identified dopamine receptor subtypes on the different aspects of sexual behavior, mainly penile erection and copulatory behavior, in order to provide an updated picture of the last discoveries and new possible advances useful for realizing new strategies for the treatment of erectile dysfunction or other related sexual disorders based on the modulation of the activity of central dopamine neurotransmission.

Table 2. Dopamine receptor agonists and their effect on penile erection and copulatory behavior

Dopamine receptor agonist	Dopamine receptor involved	Effect on penile erection	Effect on copulatory behavior	References
apomorphine	$D_1/D_2/D_3/D_4/D_5$	facilitatory	facilitatory	[30, 45-48, 71, 74]
quinpirole	$D_2/D_3/D_4$	facilitatory	facilitatory	[30,45]
pramipexole	D_3/D_2	facilitatory	facilitatory	[42, 43, 45, 86, 87]
PD 128,907	D_3/D_2	facilitatory	not available	[45, 46]
PNU-95666E	D_2	facilitatory	not available	[45]
PD 168,077	D_4	facilitatory	facilitatory	[36, 38, 39, 42-44, 71, 74]
ABT-724	D_4	facilitatory	facilitatory	[35, 74]
PIP3EA	D_4	facilitatory	not available	[37, 38]
FAUC 3019	D_4	facilitatory	not available	[40]
FAUC 389	D_4	facilitatory	not available	[41]
A-412997	D_4	facilitatory	not available	[78]
CP 226269	D_4	facilitatory	not available	[71]

Appropriate references are quoted in the Dopamine receptors Section.

DOPAMINE AND ERECTILE FUNCTION

As recalled above, preclinical studies have shown that dopamine influences erectile function by acting in different brain areas, which include the hypothalamic PVN, the MPOA and the NAc. Accordingly, after the pioneering work of Hull, Melis, Argiolas and coworkers, which revealed that the dopamine agonist apomorphine was able to induce penile erection when injected into the MPOA [47] and in the PVN [48], respectively, by acting on dopamine receptors of the D2 family (see below), dopamine activity was found to be increased in these areas when penile erection occurs in physiological contexts (the so called noncontact erections, which are penile erections observed in sexually potent male rats when put into the presence of an inaccessible receptive female, that the male can see, hear, smell but not touch) [49, 50] and during copulation [51]. In this regard, it is important to recall that dopamine in the hypothalamus is present in the so called incerto-hypothalamic dopaminergic neurons, which have their cell bodies in the A13 and A14 areas of Dahlstrom and Fuxe [52], arborize extensively and innervate hypothalamic nuclei as the PVN and the MPOA [53, 54], and in the tubero-infundibular dopaminergic neurons that originate in the periventricular area and project to the median eminence, in which dopamine is released in the hypophyseal portal blood system to control prolactin secretion from pituitary lactotrophs [55]. As to the mechanisms activated by the stimulation of D2-like receptors leading to penile erection, it was soon discovered that dopamine agonists induce penile erection when injected into the hypothalamic PVN by acting on receptors located in the cell bodies of oxytocinergic neurons projecting to extra-hypothalamic brain areas, such as the VTA, the hippocampus and the spinal cord, leading to the release of oxytocin in these areas, which in turn activates the erectile response (see [30, 13]). It was also found that dopamine agonist-induced penile erection occurred concomitantly to an increase in nitric oxide production in the PVN. Newly formed nitric oxide in turn activated oxytocinergic neurons to release oxytocin in the extra-hypothalamic brain areas recalled above and in the spinal cord leading to penile erection. In line with this hypothesis, nitric oxide synthase inhibitors given into the PVN before the injection of dopamine agonists, were found able to reduce nitric oxide production and penile erection. Conversely, penile erection induced by dopamine agonists injected into the PVN was also reduced by selective oxytocin receptor antagonists given into the lateral ventricles, but not into the PVN (see [17, 19, 20, 26]). The discovery that dopamine agonists activate oxytocinergic neurons projecting to the extra-hypothalamic brain area such as the VTA, led to suggest that an increased dopamine activity in the PVN can also activate mesolimbic dopaminergic neurons, thus increasing dopamine activity in the NAc, as it was found to occur during non contact erections and copulation. In line with this hypothesis, oxytocin injected into the VTA was found able to induce penile erection and to increase extracellular dopamine in the dialysate obtained from the NAc [56, 57], as found with dopamine agonists injected into the PVN [39]. Together with other findings showing that oxytocin induces penile erection also when injected into the hippocampal ventral subiculum and into the posterior nucleus of the amygdala [58] apparently by increasing the activity of mesolimbic dopaminergic neurons via an activation of glutamatergic nerve endings impinging on the cell bodies of mesolimbic dopaminergic neurons in the VTA [59, 60], these studies lead to suggest that a neural circuit connects the PVN with the VTA directly or indirectly (through the ventral subiculum and/or the posteromedial cortical nucleus of the amygdala) and the NAc, and from here through unknown pathways back again to the PVN to control the activity of oxytocinergic neurons projecting to the spinal cord mediating penile erection and of oxytocinergic neurons projecting to the VTA, the ventral subiculum and the posteromedial cortical nucleus of the amygdala, modulating in this way the activity of mesolimbic dopaminergic neurons (Figure 1) (see [20]). This complex neural circuit may play a role in the integration of neural activities involved in the control of the consummatory (erectile–ejaculatory) and anticipatory (motivational and rewarding) aspects of male sexual behavior in physiological contexts. Indeed, extracellular dopamine increases in the NAc [32] and in the paraventricular nucleus of sexually potent male rats during exposure to an inaccessible receptive female rat, when noncontact erections occur, and even more when copulation is allowed, e.g., when *in copula* penile erections occur [51]. Thus, it is reasonable to assume that this complex neural circuit, while contributing to the consummatory aspects of sexual behavior at the level of the hypothalamus, in the same time may also activate the mesolimbic dopaminergic system providing a neural substrate for explaining the rewarding properties of sexual activity [61, 32]. Indeed, the NAc is the brain area that contains the nerve endings of mesolimbic dopaminergic neurons and in which dopamine release is increased during the anticipatory and consummatory phase of sexual activity [32]. It is well known that the NAc plays a key role in motivation and reward for natural stimuli, i.e., food and sex. The rewarding properties of sexual activity are important for reproduction, as this leads animals and humans to look for and to engage themselves in sexual activity. In this regard, it is noteworthy that the mesolimbic dopaminergic system activated by dopamine agonists injected into the PVN as well as by oxytocin injected into the VTA is also activated by drugs of abuse such as opiates, cannabinoids, amphetamine, cocaine and alcohol [62].

It is likely that the above recalled neural circuit includes also the MPOA, as dopamine facilitates penile erection and sexual activity not only by acting at the level of the PVN and the NAc, but also of the MPOA. Accordingly, dopamine agonists injected into the MPOA induce penile erection, facilitate penile reflexes and ejaculation (see [33]). A facilitatory role of nitric oxide on the above functions has been also found in this area [63], as found in the PVN. Microdialysis studies have also shown that dopamine activity is increased during the anticipatory phase of sexual behavior when noncontact penile erections occur, and even more during copulation [33]. However, the neural pathways activated in the MPOA by dopamine agonists mediating the facilitatory effects on erectile function (and sexual activity), are still unknown. Interestingly, a recent study supports the hypothesis that in the MPOA also dopamine may contribute to activate oxytocinergic neurotransmission, as found in the PVN [64]. Although further studies are necessary to confirm such hypothesis, the increase of extracellular dopamine concentration found during copulation in the PVN and/or the MPOA is believed to be related mainly to sexual performance, e.g., to the consummatory phase of sexual behavior (penile erection and copulation), while that found in the NAc is considered to be related to the appetitive effects of sexual activity, but a role of the PVN and the MPOA in sexual motivation may also occur as well (see [20, 39, 56] and references therein).

DOPAMINE RECEPTORS AND ERECTILE FUNCTION

As recalled above, the characterization of several D_1-like (D_1 and D_5) and D_2-like (D_2, D_3 and D_4) receptor subtypes by molecular biology studies opened the research aimed at the identification of the dopamine receptor subtypes mediating the effect of the mixed dopamine receptor agonists on erectile response at the level of the brain areas in which these compounds act to induce penile erection. Since three receptors of the D_2 subtype (D_2, D_3 and D_4) were identified and different variants cloned (see [65-67]), it become important to identify the exact role of each one of these receptor subtypes in erectile function. Of the numerous molecules synthesized and identified for a selective effect on these dopaminergic receptors *in vitro*, only a few were found to interact with a selectivity high enough to discriminate among the D_2, D_3 and D_4 receptor subtypes when expressed in cultured transfected cells (Table 3). While many of these molecules act mainly as selective antagonists of the D_2, D_3 and D_4 receptors, it has been difficult and it is still unknown how to obtain agonists that act with high selectivity on the D_2 and the D_3 receptors, respectively (that is, compounds with a different affinity for these two receptors have been identified, but this different affinity is not high enough to allow a selective activation of only one of the two receptors without affecting also the other one).

In contrast to the lack of highly selective D_2 and D_3 receptor agonists, molecules that act as agonists of the D_4 receptor subtype selective enough to allow the stimulation of D_4 receptors without acting on D_2 and D_3 receptors, have been identified (see Table 3).

Table 3. Binding affinities of the D_2-like agonists and antagonists used in *in vitro* studies on the D_2, D_3, and D_4 receptors

Dopaminergic drugs	Binding affinities at			References
	D_2 receptors	D_3 receptors	D_4 receptors	
	Ki values (nM)			
Agonists				
apomorphine	32	26	2.6	[71]
quinpirole	1.8	0.96	3.0	[81]
pramipexole	3.9	0.5	5.1	[81]
PD 128,907	931	9.7	2430	[45]
PNU-95,666E	144	493	>10000	[45]
PD 168,077	3740	2810	8.7	[75]
ABT-724	>10000	NR	63.6	[35]
PIP3EA	990	3900	2.8	[37]
FAUC 3019	33	82	0.4	[40]
FAUC 389	210	390	1.5	[41]
A-412997	2848	2095	7.9	[78]
CP 226269	1760	NR	6.0	[83]
Antagonists				
L-741,626	2.4	100	220	[77]
SB277011A	1000	10	NR	[84]
FAUC 365	3600	0.5	340	[85]
L-745,870	960	2300	0.43	[77]
haloperidol	6.3	6.1	10	[80]
raclopride	1.0	1.3	5070	[82]

NR = not reported.

During one of the studies aimed at characterizing the dopamine receptor subtypes involved in the facilitatory effect of mixed dopamine receptor agonists on penile erection, ABT-724, one of these selective dopamine D_4 agonists, was found able to induce penile erection when given systemically and into the lateral ventricles to male rats, with a potency similar to that of apomorphine [35]. In agreement with the results of these studies, other D_4 agonists, such as CP 226269, PD 168,077, PIP3EA, A-412997, FAUC 3019 and FAUC 389 (Table 3), were found capable of inducing penile erection. Some of these compounds were found able to induce penile erection when given not only systemically and into the lateral ventricles, but also into the PVN, apparently by activating oxytocinergic neurons mediating penile erection with a mechanism similar to that of apomorphine and other D2-like agonists, e.g., by increasing oxytocinergic neurotransmission [29, 36-41]. Accordingly, like apomorphine, PD 168,077 injected into the PVN at doses that induce penile erection, increased nitric oxide production in the PVN dialysate obtained by intracerebral microdialysis, and this effect was antagonized by NO-synthase inhibitors given into the PVN prior the injection of the D_4 agonists at doses that reduce the D_4 agonist induced erectile response [38]. PD 168,077-induced penile erection was also abolished by omega-conotoxin GVIA, a potent blocker of voltage dependent Ca^{2+} channels given into the PVN prior the D_4 agonist, and by $d(CH_2)_5$-$Tyr(Me)^2$-Orn^8-vasotocin, a selective oxytocin receptor antagonist, given into the lateral ventricles but not into the PVN [38, 39]. Finally, like apomorphine, PD 168,077 injected into the PVN at doses that induce penile erection increased also the concentration of extracellular dopamine in the dialysate obtained by intracerebral microdialysis from the shell of the NAc [39]. Since L-745,870, a selective D_4 receptor antagonist, was found capable of abolishing PD 168,077-induced penile erection and associated responses (e.g., increased nitric oxide production in the PVN, extracellular dopamine increase in the dialysate obtained from the NAc) [36, 38, 39] and functional D_4 receptors are present in the PVN together with D_2 and D_3 receptor subtypes, being all located in the cell bodies of oxytocinergic neurons in the PVN [28, 29, 68], these studies lead to suggest that dopamine agonists induce penile erection by acting mainly on D_4 receptors [35]. Finally, since some of these D_4 agonists, unlike apomorphine, were found ineffective in inducing emesis in the ferret, a classic animal model of emesis in mammals [69, 70], this reopened the research on dopamine agonists that induce penile erection but devoid of the collateral emetic effects of classic dopamine agonists.

The unavailability of highly selective agonists of the receptors of the D_2 and D_3 subtype lead to study the effect of the available D_2, D_3 and D_4 receptor preferring antagonists (i.e., L-741,626, SB277011A, FAUC 365, L-745,870 and others) on the erectile response induced by the mixed dopamine receptor agonists such as apomorphine, quinpirole, quinelorane and pramipexole, and by the D_3 receptor preferring agonist PD-128,907 and D_4 receptor agonists (ABT-724, PD 168,077, PIP3EA, CP 226269 and others), in order to provide further evidence that these compounds induce penile erection in male rats by acting mainly on D_4 receptors. Unexpectedly, the first two of these studies produced conflicting results. Indeed, while the first study showed a main role of D_3 receptors in mediating penile erection induced by the mixed dopamine receptors agonists apomorphine and pramipexole [45], the second provided evidence for a main role of D_2 receptors [46]. The main role of D_3 receptors supported by the first study was attributed by the Authors of the second study, to the ability of the putative D_3 receptor antagonists used in the first study, S33084 and SB277011A, to reduce the proerectile response induced by the mixed dopamine agonists apomorphine and pramipexole, because these were used at doses high enough to block not only D_3 but also D_2 receptors (see [46]). Perhaps more important for this review, both these studies failed to find a proerectile effect of D_4 agonists in rats against the results of the studies quoted above showing a proerectile effect of D_4 receptor agonists. The reason for these different results is unknown and difficult to explain, also in view of the very similar experimental procedures and compounds used in these two studies and in the previous studies. In order to spread some light on these contrasting results, we have done studies similar to those described in the above studies in our laboratory [42, 43]. Briefly, the effect of L-741,626, a selective D_2 antagonist, raclopride, a D_2/D_3 antagonist, SB277011A and FAUC 365, two selective D_3 antagonists, L-745,870, a selective D_4 antagonist, and haloperidol, a classical antagonist of all D2-like-receptors, given systemically or directly into the PVN (e.g., one of the brain areas where dopamine agonists act to induce penile erection, see Introduction), respectively, on penile erection induced by apomorphine and pramipexole, which stimulate both D_2, D_3 and D_4 receptors, given systemically or directly into the PVN in male rats, respectively, was studied (Figure 2).

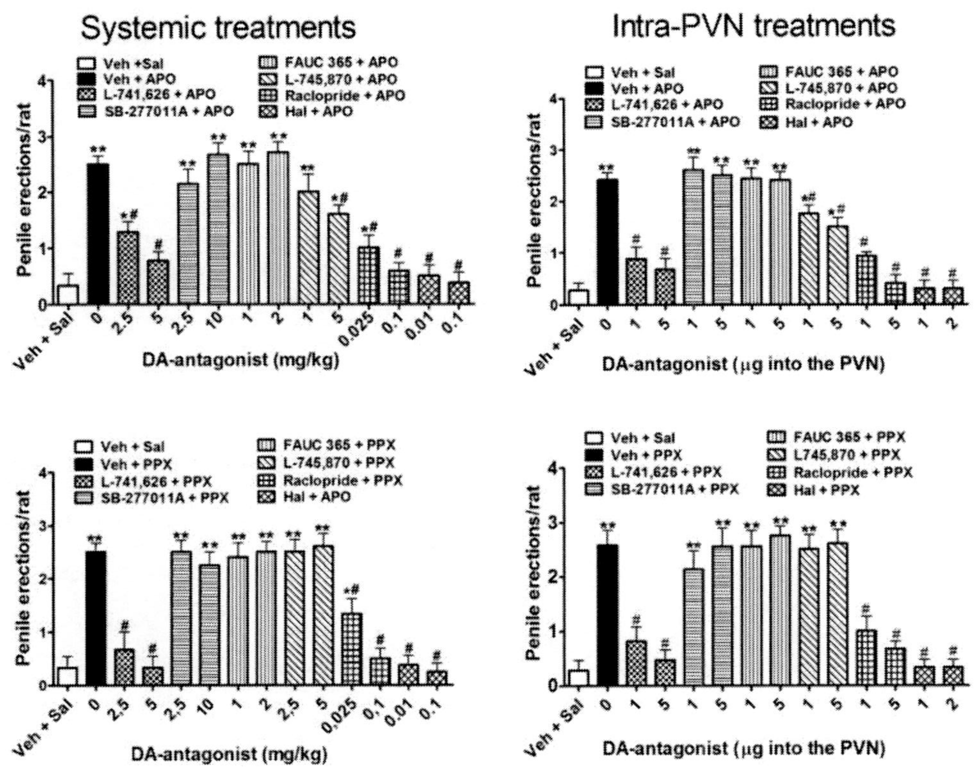

Figure 2. Effect of selective and non selective D_2, D_3 and D_4 receptor antagonists on penile erection induced by apomorphine and pramipexole. (Continued)

Briefly L-741,626, a selective D_2 antagonist, raclopride, a D_2/D_3 antagonist, SB277011A and FAUC 365, two selective D_3 antagonists, L-745,870, a selective D_4 antagonist, and haloperidol, a classical antagonist of all D2-like receptors, were given subcutaneously (in a volume of 0.2 ml/200 g body weight of appropriate vehicle 15 min before the dopamine agonists) or directly into the PVN (in a volume of 0.5 μl of appropriate vehicle before the dopamine agonists through chronic guide cannulas aimed at the PVN implanted under isoflurane anaesthesia seven days before the experiments), respectively, on penile erection induced by apomorphine and pramipexole given either subcutaneously in a volume of 0.2 ml/200 g body weight of appropriate vehicle (0.08 mg/kg and 0.1 mg/kg, of apomorphine and pramipexole, respectively) or directly into the PVN in a volume of 0.5 μl of saline in male rats (50 ng of each drug), respectively. Penile erections were counted by an observer who was not aware of the treatments. Values are means ± SEM of 8 rats/group. * $P < 0.05$, ** $P < 0.01$ with respect to vehicle treated rats; # $P < 0.05$ with respect to the corresponding group treated with DA agonist alone (one-way ANOVA followed by Bonferroni's pair wise post hoc contrasts).

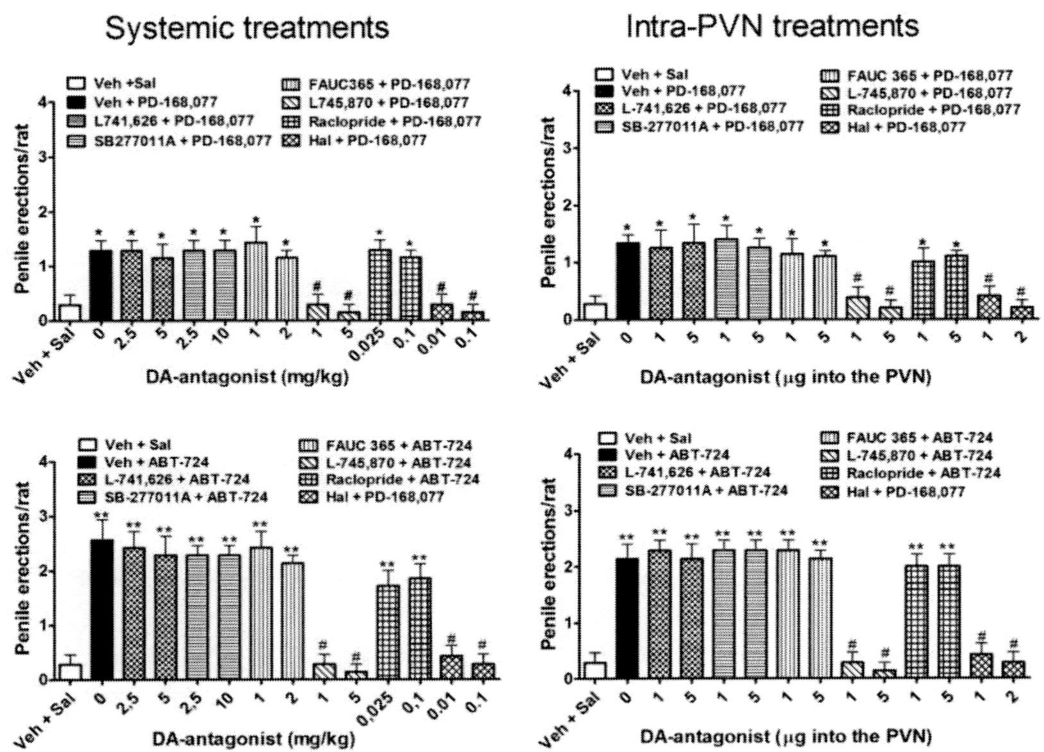

Figure 3. Effect of selective and non selective D_2, D_3 and D_4 receptor antagonists on penile erection induced by the D_4 receptcr agonists PD 168,077 and ABT-724. (Continued)

Briefly L-741,626, a selective D_2 receptor antagonist, raclopride, a D_2/D_3 receptor antagonist, SB277011A and FAUC 365, two selective D_3 receptor antagonists, L-745,870, a selective D_4 receptor antagonist, and haloperidol, a classic antagonist of all D2-like receptors, were given subcutaneously (in a volume of 0.2 ml/200 g body weight of appropriate vehicle 15 min before the dopamine D_4 agonists) or directly into the PVN (in a volume of 0.5 µl of appropriate vehicle before the dopamine D_4 agonists through chronic guide cannulas aimed at the PVN implanted under isoflurane anaesthesia seven days before the experiments), respectively, on penile erection induced by PD 168,077 and ABT-724 given either subcutaneously in a volume of 0.2 ml/200 g body weight of saline (0.1 mg/kg of PD 168,077 and 0.04 mg/kg of ABT-724) or directly into the PVN in a volume of 0.5 µl of saline in male rats, (0.1 µg of PD 168,077 and 0.05 µg of ABT-724), respectively. Penile erections were counted for 60 min by an observer who was not aware of the treatments. Values are means ± SEM of 8 rats/group. * $P < 0.05$, ** $P < 0.01$ with respect to vehicle treated rats; # $P< 0.05$ with respect to the corresponding group treated with DA agonist alone (one-way ANOVA followed by Bonferroni's pair wise post hoc contrasts).

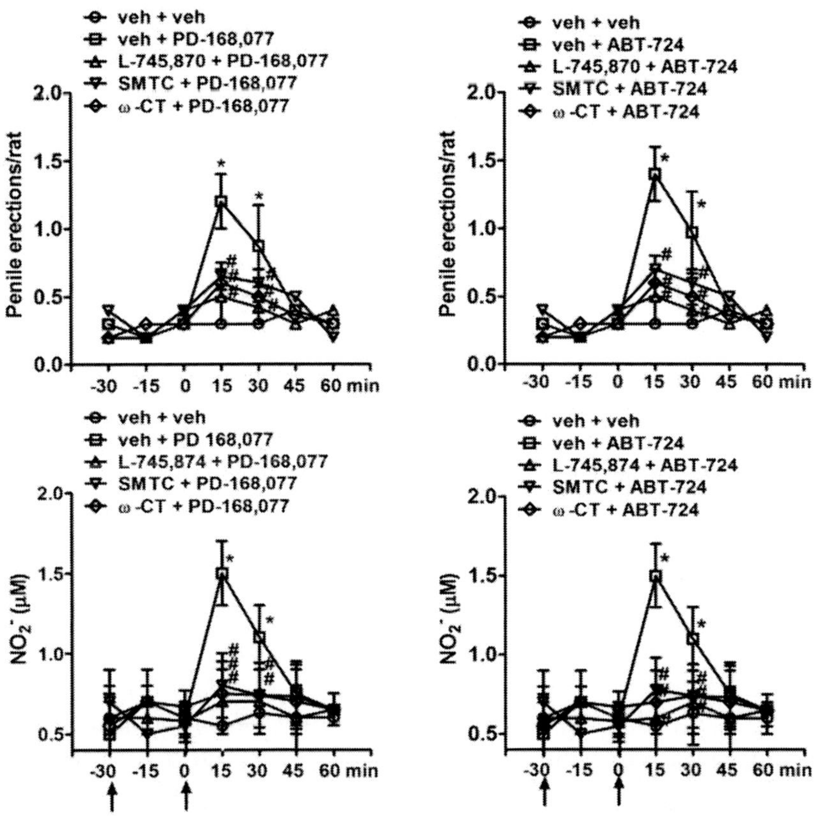

Figure 4. Intra-PVN PD 168,077- and ABT-724-induced penile erection and increase in NO production in the PVN dialysate of male rats: reversal by intra PVN injections of L-745,870, SMTC and ω-CT. Briefly, L-745,870 (1 μg), SMTC (20 μg) and ω-CT (5 ng) were given into the PVN in a volume of 0.5 μl of appropriate vehicle 30 min before the D_4 agonists of male rats stereotaxically implanted with a microdialysis probe directed at and associated to a microinjection cannula directed to the PVN and already perfused for 1 hr in order to equilibrate the extracellular fluid with the dialysis buffer. PD 168,077(0.1 μg) and ABT-724 (0.05 μg) were given into the PVN in a volume of 0.5 μl of appropriate vehicle. Penile erections were counted for 60 min by an observer who was not aware of the treatments. Dialysate aliquots were collected and nitrite (NO_2^-) concentration measured as an index of nitric oxide production in the PVN (see [88]). Values are means ± SEM of 8 rats/group. * $P < 0.05$ with respect to vehicle treated rats; # $P< 0.05$ with respect to the corresponding group treated with D_4 agonist alone (two-way ANOVA followed by Bonferroni's pair wise post hoc contrasts).

The results of these experiments are in line with the hypothesis that D_2 rather than D_3 receptors mediate the proerectile effect of these mixed non selective dopamine receptor agonists either when given systemically or when given into the PVN. Accordingly the proerectile effect of both apomorphine and pramipexole was antagonized by the prior administration of D_2 but not D_3 receptor antagonists. These experiments also showed that the proerectile effect of pramipexole given systemically or into the PVN was not antagonized by the D_4 antagonist L-745,870, also given systemically or into the PVN, although this compound caused a decrease of about 30% of the proerectile effect of apomorphine, either after systemic or intra-PVN administration of the two drugs, as already reported in previous studies (see [38, 39]). These findings raise the possibility that D_4 receptors may have some role, although modest, in the proerectile effect of apomorphine, but not of pramipexole.

Against the results of the above two studies that failed to find a pro-erectile effect of D_4 receptor agonists [45, 46], and again in line with those of previous studies showing a proerectile effect of D_4 receptor agonists in male rats, our results confirmed definitively that the two D_4 receptor agonists PD 168,077 and ABT-724 induce penile erection either when given systemically or into the PVN, with ABT-724 and PD 168,077 showing the first a potency similar to and the second lower than that of apomorphine and pramipexole (Figure 3).

As expected, and in line with the results of previous studies with PD 168,077 [35-38, 43, 44], the proerectile effect of these two D_4 agonists was completely abolished by the D_4 receptor antagonist L-745,870, but not by the D_2 receptor antagonist L-741,626, the D_2/D_3 receptor antagonist raclopride or the D_3 receptor antagonists SB277011A and FAUC 365, given either systemically or into the PVN prior of the D_4 receptor agonists (Figure 3). These results, and in particular the ability of these two D_4 agonists to induce penile erection when given into the PVN, suggest that the selective stimulation of D_4 receptors in the PVN, is sufficient per se to induce penile erection.

Since D_4 receptors are located in the cell bodies of oxytocinergic neurons (see [28, 29] and are apparently coupled to a G-protein that allows the increase in Ca^{2+} influx in these cell bodies [68], these finding are in line with the hypothesis that the stimulation of these D_4 receptors induces penile erection by activating oxytocinergic neurons projecting to the spinal cord and to extra-hypothalamic brain areas as already shown for the stimulation of D_2 receptors by apomorphine (see above) [13, 17, 20, 30, 38, 39]. Accordingly, penile erection induced by PD 168,077 and ABT-724 occurred concomitantly to an increase in nitric oxide production in the PVN, as measured by the increased concentration of nitrites in the dialysate obtained from the PVN by intracerebral microdialysis (Figure 4).

Both these responses (penile erection and increased nitric oxide production in the PVN dialysate) were abolished by the prior injection into the PVN not only of L-745,847, that blocks D_4 receptors, but also of S-methyl-thiocitrulline, an inhibitor of neuronal Ca^{2+}-calmodulin dependent nitric oxide synthase, that converts L-arginine to nitric oxide, and of omega-conotoxin GVIA, a potent inhibitor of voltage-dependent Ca^{2+} channels. That the increase in nitric oxide production in the PVN induced by the stimulation of D_4 receptors causes the activation of oxytocinergic neurons mediating penile erection is further supported by the findings showing that the potent and selective oxytocin receptor antagonist $d(CH_2)_5Tyr(Me)^2$-Orn^8-vasotocin given into the lateral ventricles but not directly into the PVN, reduces almost completely PD 168,077- and ABT-724-induced penile erection without reducing the concomitant increase in nitric oxide production (Figure 5).

Together, the results of the above studies support the hypothesis that D_4 receptor agonists induce penile erection by activating mechanisms similar to those activated by the stimulation of D_2 receptors, although with a potency lower than that of mixed dopamine receptor agonists, such as apomorphine and quinpirole [42, 43]. Such lower potency of D_4 receptor agonists in facilitating penile erection may be due to the higher affinity of apomorphine and quinpirole for D_4 receptors when compared to PD 168,077 and ABT-724, as suggested by in vitro studies showing that 1) the EC50 of apomorphine (6.0 nM) and quinpirole (60 nM) is much lower than that of PD 168,077 (83 nM) and ABT-724 (281 nM) in increasing the GTPγS binding activity in CHO cells transfected with human D_4 receptors (e.g., a measure of the activation of G-protein coupled receptors after receptor binding, which is used to study the activation of D_4 receptors [71-73]), and 2) the maximal efficacy of apomorphine (84%) and quinpirole (95%) is higher than that of PD 168,077 (68%) and ABT-724 (61%) when compared to dopamine (100%) in increasing Ca^{2+} influx in HEK-293 cells co-transfected with rat/human D_4 receptors and a G protein (Gαq05) (see [70] and references therein). Alternatively, PD 168,077 and ABT-724 may act as dopamine D_4 receptor partial agonists, or the concomitant activation of different dopamine receptor subtypes by apomorphine and quinpirole may produce a higher activation of the targets (see below), which lead to penile erection, than the activation of one dopamine receptor subtype only.

Finally, D2-like receptor agonists induce penile erection, facilitate penile reflexes and ejaculation also when injected into the MPOA (see [33]).

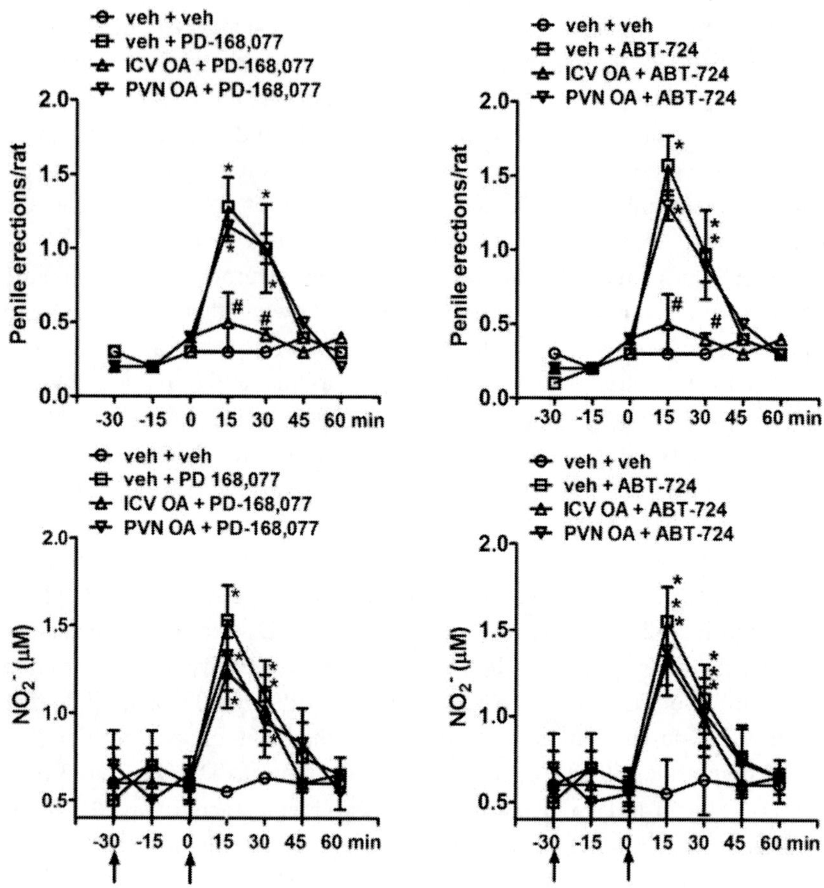

Figure 5. Intra PVN PD 168,077 and ABT-724-induced penile erection and increase in NO production in the PVN dialysate of male rats: reversal by ICV but not intra PVN oxytocin antagonist d(CH_2)$_5$-Tyr(Me)^2-Orn^8-vasotocin. Briefly, the oxytocin antagonist (1 μg) was given into the PVN in a volume of 0.5 μl or in a volume of 10 μl into the lateral ventricles 30 min before the D_4 receptor agonists of male rats stereotaxically implanted with a microdialysis probe directed at and associated with a microinjection cannula directed to the PVN or ICV and already perfused for 1 hr in order to equilibrate the extracellular fluid with the dialysis buffer. PD 168,077 (0.1 μg) and ABT-724 (0.05 μg) were given into the PVN in a volume of 0.5 μl of appropriate vehicle. Penile erections were counted for 60 min by an observer who was not aware of the treatments. Dialysate aliquots were collected and nitrite (NO_2^-) concentration measured as an index of NO production in the PVN (see [88]). Values are means ± SEM of 8 rats/group. * $P < 0.05$ with respect to vehicle treated rats; # $P < 0.05$ with respect to the corresponding group treated with D_4 receptor agonist alone (two-way ANOVA followed by Bonferroni's pair wise post hoc contrasts).

A facilitatory role of nitric oxide on the above responses has been also found in this area [63], as found in the PVN. Microdialysis studies have also shown that dopamine activity is increased when noncontact penile erections occur, and even more during copulation [33]. However, the neural pathways activated in the MPOA by dopamine mediating the facilitatory effects on erectile function and sexual activity, are still unknown. Interestingly, a recent study supports the hypothesis that also in the MPOA dopamine may contribute to activate oxytocinergic neurotransmission, as found in the PVN [64]. However, to our knowledge no study is available so far suggesting a role of D_4 receptors in the MPOA in the proerectile effect of D2-like receptor agonists.

DOPAMINE RECEPTORS AND COPULATORY BEHAVIOR

As recalled above (see Introduction), classical mixed dopamine receptor agonists, such as apomorphine, pramipexole quinpirole and quinelorane, not only facilitate penile erection in *ex copula* contexts (e.g., in the absence of any sexual stimuli, as the presence of a receptive female), but also facilitate sexual behavior of sexually potent male rats, as inferred by the changes induced in these rats in copulatory parameters measured in classical copulation tests with an ovariectomized receptive (estrogen + progesterone-primed) female rat, mainly a decrease in mount and intromission frequency and ejaculation latency, and an increase in ejaculation frequency (see [30] and references therein). In spite of the studies quoted above supporting a proerectile role of D_4 receptor agonists, to our knowledge, only one detailed study (made in the laboratory of the Authors) is available on the effect of two D_4 receptor agonists, PD 168,077 and ABT-724, given systemically, on the copulatory behavior of sexually potent male rats [74].

A comparison of the sexual effects of these two D_4 agonists with those of apomorphine is also reported. Briefly this study shows that the two D_4 receptor agonists tested facilitate copulatory behavior of sexually potent male rats as indicated by the changes in several copulatory parameters, e.g., the two compounds decreased in a dose-dependent manner mount frequency, post-ejaculatory interval and increased ejaculation frequency, without modifying significantly the other measured copulatory parameters (Table 4). Many of these changes were similar to those induced by apomorphine, except for post ejaculatory interval, which was not found to be modified by the mixed D_1/D_2 dopamine agonist, at variance from the two D_4 receptor agonists, which shortened significantly this sexual parameter.

On the other hand, apomorphine modified also other copulatory parameters, e.g., it decreased ejaculation latency and intromission frequency, which were not affected by PD 168,077 or ABT-724 (Table 4).This study showed also a comparison of the effect of L-745,870, a selective D_4 receptor antagonist, on copulatory behavior with that of haloperidol, a classic dopamine receptor antagonist that blocks all D2 receptor subtypes.

Table 4. Effect of PD 168,077 and ABT-724 on copulatory parameters (mount, intromission and ejaculation latencies and mount, intromission and ejaculation frequencies and post ejaculatory interval) of sexually potent male rats: comparison with apomorphine

Treatments	ML (sec)	IL (sec)	EL (sec)	MF (n)	IF (n)	EF (n)	PEI (sec)
Sal	50.8 ± 0.8	62.5 ± 1.2	578.5 ± 28	8.3 ± 0.7	14.9 ± 0.7	2.7 ± 0.1	381.6 ± 16.6
PD (0.05)	56.0 ± 0.6	70.2 ± 0.6	553.2 ± 29.2	7.75 ± 0.7	14.9 ± 0.9	2.8 ± 0.2	378.1 ± 18
PD (0.2)	49.5 ± 0.6	58.9 ± 0.6	538.4 ± 33.7	4.85 ± 0.4*	14.4 ± 0.8	3.5 ± 0.2*	282.0 ± 9.0*
ABT (0.01)	50.0 ± 0.7	58.1 ± 0.7	588.5 ± 23.9	4.95 ± 0.8*	13.8 ± 0.5	2.7 ± 0.2	366.0 ± 14.9
ABT (0.04)	49.1 ± 0.7	63.6 ± 1.2	398.2 ± 16.9*	3.95 ± 0.6*	14.1 ± 0.7	3.5 ± 0.2*	297.4 ± 10.5*
APO (0.02)	50.8 ± 0.8	62.5 ± 1.4	351.5 ± 26.7*	4.3 ± 0.9*	14.9 ± 0.6	3.5 ± 0.2*	361.6 ± 23.7
APO (0.08)	46.0 ± 0.5	56.0 ± 1.6	229.0 ± 22*	2.0 ± 0.2*	8.7 ± 0.4*	3.7 ± 0.3*	369.0 ± 20.8

PD 168,077 (PD) (0.05-0.2 mg/kg SC), ABT-724 (ABT) (0.01-0.04 mg/kg SC) or apomorphine (APO) (0.02-0.08 mg/kg SC) or saline alone (Sal) was given to male rats. Ten minutes after treatment, a sexually receptive female was put into the cage and the male rat was observed for 60 min in order to measure copulatory parameters. Values are means ± SEM of 10 rats per group. * $P < 0.05$ with respect to the corresponding group treated with vehicles alone (Sal) (two-way ANOVA followed by Bonferroni's pair wise post hoc contrasts).

In line with the facilitatory effect exerted by the selective stimulation of D_4 receptors by the two D_4 receptor agonists on male copulatory behavior, L-745,870 impaired copulatory behavior of sexually potent male rats, as measured by the changes induced by this D_4 receptor antagonist on several copulatory parameters. Accordingly, L-745,870 increased dose-dependently intromission and ejaculation latency, mount frequency and post ejaculatory interval, and decreased ejaculation frequency (Table 5). These changes are similar to those found with haloperidol, although the latter drug induced changes in almost all the copulatory parameters measured as expected, including those not affected by the D_4 receptor antagonist. Indeed, haloperidol was also very effective in increasing mount latency and in reducing the intromission frequency, parameters that were not modified by L-745,870 (Table 5).

Table 5. Effect of L-745,870 on copulatory parameters (mount, intromission and ejaculation latencies and mount, intromission and ejaculation frequencies and post ejaculatory interval) of sexually potent male rats: comparison with haloperidol

Treatments	ML (sec)	IL (sec)	EL (sec)	MF (n)	IF (n)	EF (n)	PEI (sec)
Sal/Veh	50.8 ± 0.8	62.5 ± 4.1	578.5 ± 23.4	8.3 ± 0.6	14.9 ± 1.1	2.7 ± 0.3	381.6 ± 23.1
L-745 (1)	62.4 ± 1.0	71.4 ± 3.2	625.5 ± 21.6	9.3 ± 0.7	15.3 ± 1.5	2.8 ± 0.5	382.3 ± 31.1
L-745 (5)	63.2 ± 1.5	183.1 ± 18.3*	991.5 ± 42.5*	13.0 ± 0.3*	14.6 ± 2.0	1.8 ± 0.2*	486.6 ± 23.1*
Hal (0.1)	70.8 ± 2.7	82.4 ± 12.6*	575.3 ± 23.3	7.0 ± 0.7	8.5 ± 0.7*	2.7 ± 0.5	351.7 ± 23.1
Hal (0.2)	210.3 ± 33.4*	354.2 ± 34.4*	1152.4 ± 42.8*	7.6 ± 0.9	7.1 ± 0.4*	2.0 ± 0.3*	479.8 ± 29.2*

L-745,870 (1-5 mg/kg IP) or haloperidol (0.1-0.2 mg/kg IP) or vehicle (saline for L-745,870 and saline with a drop of acetic acid, pH = 5.0 for haloperidol) (Sal/Veh) was given to male rats. Fifteen minutes after treatment, a sexually receptive female rat was put into the cage and the male rat was observed for 60 min in order to measure copulatory parameters. Values are means ± SEM of 10 rats per group. * $P < 0.05$ with respect to the corresponding group treated with vehicles alone (Sal) (two-way ANOVA followed by Bonferroni's pair wise post hoc contrasts).

Finally, in line with the hypothesis that PD 168,077 and ABT-724 facilitate male copulatory behavior by acting mainly on D_4 receptors, L-745,870 given prior PD 168,077 or ABT-724, abolished almost completely the facilitatory effects of both D_4 receptor agonists on copulatory parameters, without altering the facilitatory sexual responses of apomorphine (Table 6).

Table 6. Effect of the dopamine D_4 receptor antagonist L-745,870 on dopamine agonist-induced changes in the values of copulatory parameters (mount, intromission and ejaculation latencies and mount, intromission and ejaculation frequencies and post ejaculatory interval) of sexually potent male rats

Treatments	ML (sec)	IL (sec)	EL (sec)	MF (n)	IF (n)	EF (n)	PEI (sec)
Sal+ Sal	50.8 ± 8	62.5 ± 2.2	578.5 ± 21.2	8.3 ± 0.8	14.9 ± 1.1	2.7 ± 0.3	381.6 ± 23.1
Sal+ PD	49.5 ± 2.0	58.9 ± 2.0	435.4 ± 16.3	4.85 ± 0.3*	14.4 ± 1.0	3.5 ± 0.3*	282.0 ± 26.2*
L-745+ Sal	63.2 ± 2.0	183.1 ± 20	991.3 ± 43.4*#	13.0 ± 0.8*#	14.6 ± 0.8	1.8 ± 0.2*#	486.6 ± 31.3*#
L-745+ PD	52.5 ± 1.8	80.1 ± 6.7	673.7 ± 28.5§	9.75 ± 0.4#	15.0 ± 1.1	2.5 ± 0.2#	382.6 ± 119.4#§
Sal+ ABT	49.1 ± 1.2	63.6 ± 2.8	398.2 ± 13.6	3.95 ± 0.2*	14.1 ± 1.0	3.5 ± 0.5*	297.4 ± 18.5*
L-745+ ABT	61.2 ± 2.1	81.9 ± 4.2	588.4 ± 21.7§	8.1 ± 0.9#§	14.8 ± 1.2	2.7 ± 0.3#§	373.4 ± 17.6#§
Sal+ APO	46.0 ± 1.3	61.0 ± 2.9	229.0 ± 11.8*	2.0 ± 0.2*	8.7 ± 0.6*	3.7 ± 0.6*	399.0 ± 21.7
L-745+ APO	56.0 ± 2.4	73.7 ± 2.8*§	356 ± 16.9*§	5.4 ± 0.4#§	9.0 ± 0.8*§	3.6 ± 0.3*§	441.4 ± 34.3

L-745,870 (L-745) (5 mg/kg IP) or saline alone (Sal) was given to male rats 15-20 min before PD 168,077 (PD) (0.2 mg/kg SC), ABT-724 (ABT) (0.04 mg/kg SC) or apomorphine (APO) (0.08 mg/kg SC) or saline alone (Sal). Ten minutes after the second treatment, a sexually receptive female was put into the cage and the male rat was observed for 60 min in order to measure copulatory parameters. Values are means ± SEM of 10 rats per group. * $P < 0.05$ with respect to the corresponding group treated with vehicles alone (Sal + Sal); # $P < 0.05$ with respect to the corresponding group treated with S + dopamine agonist (PD, ABT, APO); § $P < 0.05$ when comparing L-745 + DA agonist-treated rats with the corresponding L-745 + Sal-treated rats (two-way ANOVA followed by Bonferroni's pair wise post hoc contrasts).

CONCLUSION

The results of the experiments shown in the chapter and of the studies reviewed above confirm that the stimulation of central dopamine receptors of the D_2 and D_4 subtypes induces penile erection in sexually potent male rats in *ex copula* conditions as well as in *in copula* conditions, i.e., when copulation is allowed. The main role of D_2 receptors in inducing penile erection and facilitating copulatory behavior of sexually potent male rats has been inferred at the moment only by studying the inhibitory effect of relatively selective D_2 and D_3 receptor antagonists on penile erection and copulatory behavior induced by mixed dopamine receptor agonists as apomorphine and pramipexole, rather than by the facilitatory effect of selective D_2 receptor agonists on penile erection and on copulatory behavior or the lack of facilitatory effect of selective D_3 receptor agonists on these behavioral responses, due the lack of D_2 or D_3 receptor agonists selective enough that would allow a clear identification of the role of these two receptor subtypes in these sexual responses. On the other hand, it is experimentally confirmed and documented that the selective stimulation of D_4 receptors (at least with PD 168,077 or ABT-724 given systemically or into the PVN) induces either penile erection in *ex copula* contexts and facilitates copulatory behavior of sexually potent male rats. This is further supported by the abolishment of the facilitatory effects of the two D_4 receptor agonists on penile erection and copulatory behavior by the prior administration of L-745,870, a selective D_4 receptor antagonist. However, despite the similarity of the sexual effects of D_4 receptor agonists with those of the dopamine mixed D_2-like receptor agonists, a few differences are evident that deserve some comment. First, the selective stimulation of D_4 receptors induces penile erection and facilitates copulatory behavior with an efficacy lower than that of mixed D_2-like dopamine agonists, such as apomorphine. The reason for such difference is unknown. As discussed above, one possibility may be that mixed D2-like dopamine agonists interact with an higher affinity on dopamine D_4 receptors when compared to PD 168,077 and ABT-724, as suggested by in vitro studies in cultured cell (see [70-73] and references therein). Alternatively, PD 168,077 and ABT-724 may act as dopamine D_4 receptor partial agonists, or the concomitant activation of different dopamine receptor subtypes by apomorphine or pramipexole may produce a higher activation of the targets, which lead to penile erection and copulation, than the activation of one dopamine receptor subtype only. Second, although haloperidol, that block all D_2-like receptors, was more effective than L-745,870 in reducing copulatory behavior of sexually potent male rats, the blockade of D_4 receptors by L-745,870, given at the highest dose used in this study showed a tendency to reduce the number of rats showing intromission and ejaculation in the first series of copulatory activity. Although not significant (possibly due to the relatively low number of rats per group used in the test), this effect did not occur with haloperidol, which was almost ineffective on this parameter when compared to vehicle at the doses used in this study.

The tendency of L-745,870 to reduce the number of rats showing intromission and ejaculation occurred in spite of the fact that all male rats treated with the D_4 receptor antagonist showed mounting with the receptive female. One explanation of this finding is that the selective blockade of D_4 receptors by L-745,870 may interfere with the expression of penile erection in *in copula* conditions. In this regard, it is noteworthy that L-745,870 was also found able to reduce not only the number of *ex copula* penile erections induced by apomorphine and pramipexole by about 30% in male rats [36, 38, 42, 43], but also the percent of rats which showed intromission when put with a receptive female for a period of 15 min when given ICV [29].

Finally, at variance with mixed dopamine receptor agonists, such as apomorphine, ABT-724 and PD 168,077 have been found unable to induce vomiting in the ferret, a classic emesis model for identifying compounds that induce nausea and vomiting [35, 69, 70]. In this regard, it is noteworthy that apomorphine, the first dopaminergic drug become commercially available for the therapy of erectile dysfunction, obtained very scarce success especially when compared to that of orally active phosphodiesterase type V inhibitors (i.e., sildenafil, vardenafil and tadalafil). This may be due to the fact that apomorphine, like other mixed D_1/D_2 receptor agonists, causes nausea and vomiting incompatible with sexual intercourse, due to the stimulation of D_2 receptors present in the chemo-trigger zone of the medulla oblongata (see [15]).

As no data is available to our knowledge on the efficacy of selective D_4 receptor agonists to induce penile erection in humans, the results presented in this chapter together with those of the other studies reviewed, provide evidence for a new possible advance in the field of dopamine and sexual behavior, that is, it would be worthwhile to test compounds that act selectively on D_4 receptors devoid of emetic properties on erectile function in humans. Although it is difficult to believe that centrally acting drugs may overcome the success of orally active phosphodiesterase inhibitors that act locally at penile level, it may be that D_4 receptor agonists represent a valuable alternative strategy for the treatment of human erectile dysfunctions.

ACKNOWLEDGMENTS

This work was partially supported by a grant from the Fondazione del Banco di Sardegna (FBS) (Prot. U68.2015/AI.61.RP) to AA, and a grant from the University of Cagliari (CAR 2014) to AA and MRM and a Master and Back 2010-2011 grant from the Autonomous Region of Sardinia)(ARS) (Code no. PRR-MAB-A2011-19138) to FS.

REFERENCES

[1] Sachs, B. D., (1978). Conceptual and neural mechanisms of masculine copulatory behavior. In: McGill T. E., Dewsbury, D. A., Sachs B. D. (Eds.), *Sex and behavior: Status and prospectus*. Plenum, New York, pp. 267-295.

[2] Bitran, D., Hull, E. M., (1987). Pharmacological analysis of male sexual behavior. *Neurosci. Biobehav. Rev.* 11, 365-389.

[3] Sachs, B. D., Meisel, R. L., (1988). The physiology of male sexual behavior. In: Knobil, E., Neil, J. (Eds.), *The Physiology of Reproduction,* Vol. 2. Raven Press, New York, pp. 1393-1485.

[4] Meisel, R. L., Sachs, B. D., (1994). The physiology of male sexual behaviour. In: Knobil, E., Neil, J. (Eds.), *The Physiology of Reproduction,* Vol. 2, second edition, Raven Press, New York, pp. 3-96.

[5] Hull, E. M., Meisel, R. L., Sachs, B. D., (2002). Male sexual behavior. In Pfaff, D. W., Arnold, A. P., Etgen, A. M., Fahrbach, S. E., Rubin, R. T. (Eds), *Hormones, Brain and Behavior,* Academic Press, New York, pp. 3-137.

[6] Caggiula, A. R., Shaw, D. H., Antelman, M., Edwards, D. J., (1976). Interactive effects of brain catecholamines and variations in sexual and non-sexual arousal on copulatory behavior of male rats. *Brain Res.* 111, 321-36.

[7] Caggiula, A. R., Herndon, J. G. Jr, Scanlon, R., Greenstone, D., Bradshaw, W., Sharp, D., (1979). Dissociation of active from immobility components of sexual behavior in female rats by central 6-hydroxydopamine: implications for CA involvement in sexual behavior and sensorimotor responsiveness. *Brain Res.* 172, 505-520.

[8] Balthazart, J., Reid, J., Absil, P., Foidart, A., Ball, G. F., (1995). Appetitive as well as consummatory aspects of male sexual behavior in

quail are activated by androgens and estrogens. *Behav. Neurosci.* 109, 485-501.

[9] Lue, T., Tanagho, E., (1987). Physiology of erection and pharmacological management of impotence. *J. Urol.* 137, 829-836.

[10] Burnett, A. L., Lowenstein, C. J., Bredt, D. S., Chang. T. S. K. and Snyder, S. H., (1992). Nitric oxide: a physiological mediator of penile erection. *Science* 257, 401-403.

[11] Rajfer, J., Aronson, W. J., Bush, P. A., Dorey, F. J., Ignarro, L. J. (1992). Nitric oxide as a mediator of relaxation of the corpus cavernosum in response to nonadrenergic, noncholinergic neurotransmission. *New England J. Med.* 326, 90-94.

[12] Andersson, J. E., Wagner, G., (1995). Physiology of erection. *Physiol. Rev.* 75, 191-236.

[13] Argiolas, A., Melis, M. R., (1995). Neuromodulation of penile erection: an overview of the role of neurotransmitters and neuropeptides. *Prog. Neurobiol.* 47, 235-255.

[14] Andersson, K. E., (2001). Pharmacology of penile erection. *Pharmacol. Rev.* 53, 417-450.

[15] Argiolas, A., (2005). Male erectile dysfunction: chemical pharmacology of penile erection. *Drug Disc. Today: Ther. Strategies* 2, 31-36.

[16] Argiolas, A., Melis, M. R., (2012). Pharmacological strategies for the therapy of erectile dysfunction. In: Grant, P.S. (Ed.), *Erectile Dysfunction: causes, risk and management.* Nova Publishers Inc., New York, U.S.A., pp. 199-334.

[17] Argiolas, A., Melis, M. R., (2005). Central control of penile erection: role of the paraventricular nucleus of the hypothalamus. *Prog. Neurobiol.* 76, 1-21.

[18] McKenna, K. E., (2000). Some proposals regarding the organization of the central nervous system control of penile erection. *Neurosci. Biobehav. Rev.* 24, 535-540.

[19] Melis, M. R., Argiolas, A., (2003). Central oxytocinergic neurotransmission: a drug target for the therapy of psychogenic erectile dysfunction. *Curr. Drugs Target* 4, 55-66.

[20] Melis, M. R., Argiolas, A., (2011). Central control of penile erection: a re-visitation of the role of oxytocin and its interaction with dopamine and glutamic acid in male rats. *Neurosci. Biobehav. Rev.* 35, 939-955.

[21] Bertolini, A., Gessa, G. L., (1981). Behavioural effects of ACTH and MSH peptides. *J. Endocrinol. Inv.* 4, 241-251.

[22] Pfaus, J. G., Gorzalka, B. B., (1987). Opioids and sexual behavior. *Neurosci Biobehav Rev.* 11, 1-34.

[23] Dornan, W. A.; Malsbury, C. W., (1989). Neuropeptides and male sexual behavior. *Neurosci. Biobehav. Rev.* 13, 1-15.

[24] Argiolas, A. (1999). Neuropeptides and sexual behavior. *Neurosci. Biobehav Rev.* 23, 1127-1142.

[25] Argiolas, A., Melis, M. R., (2013). Neuropeptides and central control of sexual behaviour from the past to the present: a review. *Prog. Neurobiol.* 108, 80-107.

[26] Argiolas, A., Melis, M. R., (2004). The role of oxytocin and the paraventricular nucleus in the sexual behaviour of male mammals. *Physiol. Behav.* 83, 309-317.

[27] Andersson, K. E., (2011). Mechanisms of penile erection and basis for pharmacological treatment of erectile dysfunction. *Pharmacol. Rev.* 63, 811-859.

[28] Baskerville, T. A., Douglas, A. J., (2008). Interaction between dopamine and oxytocin in the control of sexual behaviour. *Prog. Brain Res.* 170, 277-289.

[29] Baskerville, T. A., Allard, J., Wayman, C., Douglas, A. J., (2009). Dopamine-oxytocin interaction in penile erection. *Eur. J. Neurosci.* 30, 2151-2164.

[30] Melis, M. R., Argiolas, A., (1995). Dopamine and sexual behaviour, *Neurosci. Biobehav. Rev.* 19, 19-38.

[31] Pfaus, J. G., Phillips, A. G., (1991). Role of dopamine in anticipatory and consummatory aspects of sexual behavior in the male rat. *Behav. Neurosci.* 105, 727-743.

[32] Pfaus, J. G., Everitt, B. J., (1995). The psychopharmacology of sexual behavior. In: Knobil, F. E., Kupfer, D. J. (Eds.), *Psychopharmacology: the fourth generation of progress*, Raven Press, New York, pp. 742-758.

[33] Hull, E. M., Du, J., Lorrain, D. S., Matuszewich, L., (1995). Extra-cellular dopamine in the medial preoptic area: implications for sexual motivation and hormonal control of copulation. *J. Neurosci.* 15, 7465-7471.

[34] Paredes, R. G., Agmo, A., (2004). Has dopamine a physiological role in the control of sexual behavior? A critical review of the evidence. *Prog. Neurobiol.* 73, 179-226.

[35] Brioni, J. D., Moreland, R. B., Cowart, M., Hsieh, G. C., Stewart, A. O., Hedlund, P., Donnelly-Roberts, D. L., Nakane, M., Lynch, J. J. 3rd, Kolasa, T., Polakowski, J. S., Osinski, M. A., Marsh, K., Andersson, K.

E., Sullivan, J. P., (2004). Activation of dopamine D_4 receptors by ABT-724 induces penile erection in rats. *Proc. Natl. Acad. Sci., USA* 101, 6758-6763.

[36] Melis, M. R., Succu, S., Mascia, M. S., Argiolas, A., (2005). PD 168,077, a selective dopamine D_4 receptor agonist, induces penile erection when injected into the paraventricular nucleus of male rats. *Neurosci. Lett.* 379, 59-62.

[37] Enguehard-Gueiffier, C., Hübner, H., El Hakmaoui, A., Allouchi, H., Gmeiner, P., Argiolas, A., Melis, M. R., Gueiffier, A., (2006). 2-[(4-phenylpiperazin-1-yl) methyl]imidazo(di)azines as selective D4-ligands. Induction of penile erection by 2-[4-(2-methoxyphenyl)piperazin-1-ylmethyl] imidazo [1,2-a]pyridine (PIP-3EA), a potent and selective D4 partial agonist. *J. Med. Chem.* 49, 3938-3947.

[38] Melis, M. R., Succu, S., Sanna, F., Mascia, M. S., Melis, T., Enguehard-Gueiffier, C., Hubner, H., Gmeiner, P., Gueiffier, A., Argiolas, A., (2006). PIP3EA and PD 168077, two selective dopamine D4 receptor agonists, induce penile erection in male rats: site and mechanism of action in the brain. *Eur. J. Neurosci.* 24, 2021-2030.

[39] Succu, S., Sanna, F., Melis, T., Boi, A., Argiolas, A., Melis, M. R., (2007). Stimulation of dopamine receptors in the paraventricular nucleus of the hypothalamus of male rats induces penile erection and increases extra-cellular dopamine in the nucleus accumbens: involvement of central oxytocin. *Neuropharmacology* 52, 1034-1043.

[40] Löber, S., Tschammer, N., Hübner, H., Melis, M. R., Argiolas, A., Gmeiner, P., (2009). The azulene framework as a novel bioisostere: design of potent dopamine D4 receptor ligands inducing penile erection. *Chem. Med. Chem.* 4, 325-328.

[41] Löber, S., Hübner, H., Buschauer, A., Sanna, F., Argiolas, A., Melis, M. R., Gmeiner, P., (2012) Novel azulene derivatives for the Treatment of Erectile Dysfunction. *Bioorg. Med. Chem. Lett.* 22, 7151-7154.

[42] Sanna, F., Succu, S., Hübner, H., Gmeiner, P., Argiolas, A., Melis, M. R., (2011). Dopamine D2-like receptor agonists induce penile erection in male rats: differential role of D_2, D_3 and D_4 receptors in the paraventricular nucleus of the hypothalamus. *Behav. Brain Res.* 225, 169-176.

[43] Sanna, F., Succu, S., Melis, M. R., Argiolas, A., (2012). Dopamine agonist-induced penile erection and yawning: differential role of D2 receptor subtypes and correlation with nitric oxide production in the

paraventricular nucleus of the hypothalamus of male rats. *Behav. Brain Res.* 230, 355-364.

[44] Sanna, F., Corda, M. G., Melis, M. R., Piludu, M. A., Löber, S., Hübner, H., Gmeiner, P., Argiolas, A., Giorgi, O., (2013). Dopamine agonist-induced penile erection and yawning: a comparative study in outbred Roman high- and low-avoidance rats. *Pharmacol. Biochem. Behav.* 109, 59-66.

[45] Collins, G. T., Truccone, A., Haji-Abdi, F., Newman A. H., Grundt, P., Rice, K. C., Husbands, S. M., Greedy, B. M., Enguehard-Gueiffer C, Gueiffer, A., Chen, J., Wang, S., Katz, J. L., Grandy, D. K., Sunahara, R. K., Woods, J. H., (2009). Proerectile effects of dopamine D2-like agonists are mediated by the D3 receptor in rats and mice. *J. Pharmacol. Exp. Ther.* 329, 210-217.

[46] Depoortère, R., Bardin, L., Rodrigues, M., Abrial, E., Aliaga, M, Newman-Tancredi, A., (2009). Penile erection and yawning induced by dopamine D_2-like receptor agonists in rats: influence of strain and contribution of dopamine D_2, but not D_3 and D_4 receptors. *Behav. Pharmacol.* 20, 303-311.

[47] Hull, E. M., Bitran, D., Pehek, E. A., Warner, R. K., Band, L. C., Holmes, G. M., (1986). Dopaminergic control of male sex behavior in rats: effects of an intracerebrally-infused agonist. *Brain Res.* 370, 73-81.

[48] Melis, M. R., Argiolas, A., Gessa, G. L., (1987). Apomorphine-induced penile erection and yawning: site of action in brain. *Brain Res.* 415, 98-104.

[49] Sachs, B. D., Akasofu, K., Citro, J. K., Daniels, S. B., Natoli, J. H., (1994). Non-contact stimulation from estrus females evokes penile erection in rats. *Physiol. Behav.* 55, 1073-1079.

[50] Sachs, B. D., (1997). Erection evoked in male rats by airborne scent from estrous females. *Physiol. Behav.* 62, 921-924.

[51] Melis, M. R., Succu, S., Mascia, M. S., Cortis, L., Argiolas, A., (2003). Extra-cellular dopamine increases in the paraventricular nucleus of male rats during sexual activity. *Eur. J. Neurosci.* 17, 1266-1272.

[52] Dahlström, A., Fuxe, K., (1964). Localization of monoamines in the lower brain stem. *Experientia* 20, 398-399.

[53] Buijs, R. M., Geffard, M., Pool, C. W., Hoorneman, E. M., (1984). The dopaminergic innervation of the supraoptic and paraventricular nucleus. A light and electron microscopical study. *Brain Res.* 323, 65-72.

[54] Lindvall, O., Björklund, A., Skagerberg, G., (1984). Selective histochemical demonstration of dopamine terminal systems in rat di- and

telencephalon: new evidence for dopaminergic innervation of hypothalamic neurosecretory nuclei. *Brain Res.* 306, 19-30.

[55] MacLeod, R. M., Lehmeyer, J. E., (1973). Studies on the mechanism of the dopamine-mediated inhibition of prolactin secretion. *Endocrinology* 94, 1077-1085.

[56] Melis, M. R., Melis, T., Cocco, C., Succu, S., Sanna, F., Pillolla, G., Boi, A., Ferri, G. L., Argiolas, A., (2007). Oxytocin injected into the ventral tegmental area induces penile erection and increases extracellular dopamine in the nucleus accumbens and paraventricular nucleus of the hypothalamus of male rats. *Eur. J. Neurosci.* 26, 1026–1035.

[57] Succu, S., Sanna, F., Cocco, C., Melis, T., Boi, A., Ferri, G. L., Argiolas, A., Melis, M. R., (2008). Oxytocin induces penile erection when injected into the ventral tegmental area of male rats: role of nitric oxide and cyclic GMP. *Eur. J. Neurosci.* 28, 813-821.

[58] Melis, M. R., Succu, S., Sanna, F., Boi, A., Argiolas, A., (2009). Oxytocin injected into the ventral subiculum or the posteromedial cortical nucleus of the amygdala induces penile erection and increases extracellular dopamine in the nucleus accumbens of male rats. *Eur. J. Neurosci.* 30, 1349–1357.

[59] Melis, M. R., Succu, S., Cocco, C., Caboni, E., Sanna, F., Boi, A., Ferri, G. L., Argiolas, A., (2010). Oxytocin induces penile erection when injected into the ventral subiculum: role of nitric oxide and glutamic acid. *Neuropharmacology* 58, 1153-1160.

[60] Succu, S., Sanna, F., Argiolas, A., Melis, M. R., (2011). Oxytocin injected into the hippocampal ventral subiculum induces penile erection in male rats by increasing glutamatergic neurotransmission in the ventral tegmental area. *Neuropharmacology* 61, 181-188.

[61] Everitt, B. J., (1990). Sexual motivation: A neural and behavioural analysis of the mechanisms underlying appetitive and copulatory responses of male rats. *Neurosci. Biobehav. Rev.* 14, 217-232.

[62] Tanda, G., Pontieri, F. E., Di Chiara, G., (1997). Cannabinoid and heroin activation of mesolimbic dopamine transmission by a common mu1 opioid receptor mechanism. *Science* 276, 2048-2050.

[63] Hull, E. M., Dominguez, J. M., (2006). Getting his act together: roles of glutamate, nitric oxide, and dopamine in the medial preoptic area. *Brain Res.* 1126, 66-75.

[64] Gil, M., Bhatt, R., Picotte, K. B., Hull, E. M., (2011). Oxytocin in the medial preoptic area facilitates male sexual behavior in the rat. *Horm. Behav.* 59, 435-443.

[65] Seeman, P., Van Tol, H. H. M., (1994). Dopamine receptor pharmacology. *Trends Pharmacol. Sci.* 15, 264-270.
[66] Sokoloff, P., Schwartz, J. C., (1995). Novel dopamine receptors half a decade later. *Trends Pharmacol. Sci.* 16, 270-275.
[67] Ginqrich, J. A., Caron, M. G., (1993). Recent advances in the molecular biology of dopamine receptors. *Ann. Rev. Neurosci.* 16, 299-321.
[68] Bitner, R. S., Nikkel, A. L., Otte, S., Martino, B., Barlow, E. H., Bhatia, P., Stewart, A. O., Brioni, J. D., Decker, M. W., Moreland, R. B., (2006). Dopamine D4 receptor signaling in the rat paraventricular hypothalamic nucleus: Evidence of natural coupling involving immediate early gene induction and mitogen activated protein kinase phosphorylation. *Neuropharmacology* 50, 521-531.
[69] Osinski, M. A., Uchic, M. E., Seifert, T., Shaughnessy, T. K., Miller, L. N., Natane, M., Cox, B. F., Brioni, J. D., Moreland, R. B., (2005). Dopamine D_2, but not D_4, receptor agonists are emetogenic in ferrets. *Pharmacol. Biochem. Behav.* 81, 211-219.
[70] Brioni, J. D., Moreland, R. B., (2006). Dopamine D_4 receptors and the regulation of penile erection. *Drug. Discov. Today: Ther. Strategies* 3, 599-604.
[71] Hsieh, G. C., Hollingsworth, P. R., Martino, B., Chang, R., Terranova, M. A., O'Neill, A. B., Lynch, J. J., Moreland, R. B., Donnelly-Roberts, D.L., Kolasa, T., Mikusa, J.P., McVey, J. M., Marsh, K. C., Sullivan, J. P., Brioni, J. D., (2004). Central mechanisms regulating penile erection in conscious rats: the dopaminergic systems related to the proerectile effect of apomorphine. *J. Pharmacol. Exp. Ther.* 308, 330-338.
[72] Newmann-Tancredi, A., Cussac, D., Audinot, V., Nicolas, J. P., De Ceuninck, F., Boutin, J. A., Millan, M. J., (2002). Differential actions of antiparkinson agents at multiple classes of monoaminergic receptor. II. Agonist and antagonist properties at subtypes of dopamine D_2-like receptor and $\alpha 1/\alpha 2$-adrenoceptor. *J. Pharmacol. Exp. Ther.* 303, 805-814.
[73] Newman-Tancredi, A., Heusler, P., Martel, J. C., Ormière, A. M., Leduc, N., Cussac, D., (2008). Agonist and antagonist properties of antipsychotics at human dopamine $D_{4.4}$ receptors: G-protein activation and K^+ channel modulation in transfected cells. *Int. J. Neuropsychopharmacol.* 11, 293-307.
[74] Sanna, F., Contini, A., Melis, M. R., Argiolas, A., (2015). Role of dopamine D_4 receptors in copulatory behavior: Studies with selective D_4 agonists and antagonists. *Pharmacol. Biochem. Behav.* 137: 110-118.

[75] Glase, S. A., Akunne, H. C., Georgic, L. M., Heffner, T. G., MacKenzie, R. G., Manley, P. J., Pugsley, T. A., Wise, L. D., (1997). Substituted [(4-phenylpiperazinyl)-methyl]benzamides: selective dopamine D_4 agonists. *J. Med. Chem.* 40, 1771-1772.

[76] Heier, R. F., Dolak, L. A., Duncan, J. N., Hyslop, D. K., Lipton, M. F., Martin, L. J., Mauragis, N. A., Piercey, N. F., Nichols, N. F., Schreur, P. J., Smith, M. W., Moon, M. W., (1997). Synthesis and biological activities of (*R*)-5,6-dihydro-*N,N*-dimethyl-4*H*-imidazo[4,5,1-*ij*]quinolin-5-amine and its metabolites. *J. Med. Chem.* 40, 639-646.

[77] Kulagowski, J. J., Broughton, H. B., Curtis, N. R., Mawer, I. M., Ridgill, M. P., Baker, R., Emms, F., Freedman, S. B., Marwood, R., Patel, S., Ragan, C. I., Leeson, P. D., (1996). 3-[[4-(4-Chlorophenyl)piperazin-1-yl]-methyl]-1H-pyrrolo[2,3-b]pyridine: an antagonist with high affinity and selectivity for the human dopamine D_4 receptor. *J Med. Chem.* 39,1941-1942.

[78] Moreland, R. B., Patel, M., Hsieh, G. C., Wetter, J. M., Marsh, K., Brioni, J. D., (2005). A-412997 is a selective dopamine D4 receptor agonist in rats. *Pharmacol. Biochem. Behav.* 82, 140-147.

[79] Patel, S., Freedman, S., Chapman, K. L., Emms, F., Fletcher, A. E., Knowles, M., Marwood, R., McAllister, G., Myers, J., Curtis, N., Kulagowski, J. J., Leeson, P. D., Ridgill, M., Graham, M., Matheson, S., Rathbone, D., Watt, A. P., Bristow, L. J., Rupniak, N.M., Baskin, E., Lynch, J. J., Ragan, C. I., (1997). Biological profile of L 745,870, a selective antagonist with high affinity for the dopamine D_4 receptor. *J. Pharmacol. Exp. Ther.* 283, 636-647.

[80] Tice, M. A., Hashemi, T., Taylor, L. A., Duffy, R. A., McQuade, R. D., (1994). Characterization of the binding of SCH 39166 to the five cloned dopamine receptor subtypes. *Pharmacol. Biochem. Behav.* 49, 567-571.

[81] Mierau, J., Schneider, F. J., Ensinger, H. A., Chio, C. L., Lajiness, M. E., Huff, R. M., (1995). Pramipexole binding and activation of cloned and expressed dopamine D_2, D_3 and D_4 receptors. *Eur. J. Pharmacol.* 290, 29-36.

[82] Millan, M. J., Newman-Tancredi, A., Brocco, M., Gobert, A., Lejeune, F., Audinot, V., Rivet, J. M., Schreiber, R., Dekeyne, A., Spedding, M., Nicolas, J. P., Peglion, J. L., (1998). S 18126 ([2-[4-(2,3-dihydrobenzo[1,4]dioxin-6-yl)piperazin-1-yl methyl]indan-2-yl]), a potent, selective and competitive antagonist at dopamine D_4 receptors: an *in vitro* and *in vivo* comparison with L 745,870 (3-(4-[4-

chlorophenyl]piperazin-1-yl)methyl-1H-pyrrolo[2, 3b]pyridine) and raclopride. *J. Pharmacol. Exp. Ther.* 287, 167-186.

[83] Zorn, S. H., Jackson, E., Johnon, C., Lewis, L., Fliri, A., (1997). CP-226269 is a selective dopamine D_4 agonist. *Soc. Neurosci. Abstr.* 23:685.

[84] Reavill, C., Taylor, S. G., Wood, M. D., Ashmeade, T., Austin, N. E., Avenell, K. Y., Boyfield, I., Branch, C. L., Cilia, J., Coldwell, M. C., Hadley, M. S., Hunter, A. J., Jeffrey, P., Jewitt, F., Johnson, C. N., Jones, D. N. C., Medhurst, A. D., Middlemiss, D. N., Nash, D. J., Riley, G. J., Routledge, C., Stemp, G., Thewlis, K. M., Trail, B., Vong, A. K. K., Hagan, J. J., (2000). Pharmacological actions of a novel, high-affinity, and selective human dopamine D_3 receptor antagonist, SB277011A. *J. Pharmacol. Exp. Ther.* 294, 1154-1165.

[85] Bettinetti, L., Schlotter, K., Hubner, H., Gmeiner, P., (2002). Interactive SAR studies: rational discovery of super-potent and highly selective dopamine D_3 receptor antagonists and partial agonists. *J. Med. Chem.* 45, 4594-4597.

[86] Ferrari, F., Pelloni, F., Giuliani, D., (1993). Behavioral evidence that different neurochemical mechanisms underly stretching-yawning and penile erection induced in male rats by SND 919, a new selective D2 dopamine receptor agonist. *Psychopharmacology* 113, 172-176.

[87] Ferrari, F., Giuliani, D., (1995). Sexual attraction and copulation in male rats: effects of the dopamine agonist SND 919. *Pharmacol. Biochem. Behav.* 50, 29-34.

[88] Melis, M. R., Succu, S., Argiolas, A., (1996). Dopamine agonists increase nitric oxide production in the paraventricular nucleus of the hypothalamus: correlation with penile erection and yawning. *Eur. J. Neurosci.* 8, 2056-63.

Biographical Sketch

Name: Fabrizio Sanna

Affiliation: Department of Biomedical Sciences, Section of Neuroscience and Clinical Pharmacology, University of Cagliari, Italy

Education:

2004, Jul. Master Degree in Psychology, University of Cagliari.

2009, Jan. PhD in Neuroscience, University of Cagliari.

Address: Department of Biomedical Sciences, Section of Neuroscience and Clinical Pharmacology, University of Cagliari, Italy, Cittadella

Universitaria, S.P. Sestu-Monserrato, Km 0,700, 09042 MONSERRATO (CA, Italy), Tel: +39-070-6754330; Fax: +39-070-6754320; Email: fabrizio.sanna@unica.it

Research and Professional Experience:

Fabrizio Sanna received his PhD in Neuroscience from the University of Cagliari, Italy, in January 2009 with a thesis on: "Dopamine-oxytocin interactions in the central control of penile erection," under the scientific supervision of Prof. Antonio Argiolas.

From December 2008 to December 2009 he worked as post doctoral researcher at the Department of Medicinal Chemistry, FAU University of Erlangen-Nuremberg, Germany, under the scientific supervision of Prof. Peter Gmeiner, on a research project aimed at the identification and characterization of new selective dopamine agonists suitable for the treatment of erectile dysfunction.

In January 2010 he has won a research grant (Autonomous Region of Sardinia, RAS, LR 07/2007, "Young Researchers") for conducting a two-years research project aimed at studying in animal models in vivo the role of the different subtypes of dopamine receptor and their mechanism of action in specific brain areas which modulate erectile function at the central level, and in March 2012 he has won a three-years research grant (Autonomous Region of Sardinia, RAS, Master & Back Program, Back -2011) for a research project in continuity with the previous ones and aimed at the study of the interactions between dopamine and oxytocin existing in specific brain areas and involved in the control of erectile function and male sexual behavior.

Currently, he is Assistant Professor at the Department of Biomedical Sciences of the University of Cagliari and is the holder of a three-year research grant obtained by competitive tender from the Italian Ministry of Education, University and Research (MIUR) for a research project aimed at the characterization of neural plasticity processes involved in the acquisition of sexual experience (motivation and performance).

Currently (January, 2016), Dr. Sanna has co-authored 28 scientific articles in peer-reviewed journals, most of them on neural circuits, transmitters, mechanisms of action involved in the central control of the different aspects of male sexual behavior and pharmacological agents suitable for the therapy of psychogenic sexual disorders as well.

Professional Appointments:

2015, Oct – today. Assistant Professor, Department of Biomedical Sciences, Neuroscience and Clinical Pharmacology Section, University of Cagliari.
2012, Mar - 2015, Mar. Research Fellow, Department of Biomedical Sciences, Neuroscience and Clinical Pharmacology Section, University of Cagliari.
2010, Jan - 2012, Jan. "Young Researcher," Department of Neuroscience, University of Cagliari.
2008, Dec - 2009, Nov. Post-doc researcher, Department of Medicinal Chemistry, FAU University of Erlangen-Nurnberg, Germany.
2008, Dec, PhD, Neuroscience, University of Cagliari.

Honors:

2005 – Three years Fellowship from the Italian Ministry of Education, University and Research (MIUR) for the Doctoral School of Neuroscience.
2008 – One year Fellowship (on a competitive tender) from the Autonomous Region of Sardinia (RAS, "Paths of High Education").
2010 – Two years Research Grant (on a competitive tender) from the Autonomous Region of Sardinia (RAS, "Young Researchers").
2012 – Three years Fellowship (on a competitive tender) from the Autonomous Region of Sardinia (RAS, Master and Back Program, Edition_2011).
2015 – Three years Research Grant (on a competitive tender) from the Italian Ministry of Education, University and Research (MIUR, Scientific Independence of Young Researchers, Edition_2014).

Publications Last Three Years:

1. SANNA, F., Contini, A., Melis, M, R,, Argiolas, A., (2015). Role of dopamine D_4 receptors in copulatory behavior: Studies with selective D_4 agonists and antagonists in male rats. *Pharmacol. Behav. Biochem.* 137,. 110-118. doi: 10.1016/j.pbb.2015.08.012.
2. SANNA, F., Piludu, M. A., Corda, M. G., Melis, M. R., Giorgi, O., Argiolas, A. ,(2015). Involvement of dopamine in the differences in sexual behavior between Roman high and low avoidance rats: An

intracerebral microdialysis study. *Behav. Brain Res.*. 281,. 177-186. doi: 10.1016/j.bbr.2014.12.009.

3. SANNA, F., Piludu, M. A., Corda, M. G., Argiolas, A., Giorgi, O., Melis, M. R., (2014). Dopamine is involved in the different patterns of copulatory behaviour of Roman High and Low Avoidance rats: studies with apomorphine and haloperidol. *Pharmacol. Biochem. Behav.* 124, 211-219. doi: 10.1016/j.pbb.2014.06.012.
4. SANNA, F., Corda, M. G., Melis, M. R., Piludu, M. A., Giorgi, O., Argiolas, A., (2014). Male Roman high and low avoidance rats show different patterns of copulatory behaviour: Comparison with Sprague Dawley rats. *Physiol. Behav.*. 127, 27-36. doi: 10.1016/ j.physbeh.2014.01.002.
5. SANNA, F., Corda, M. G., Melis, M. R., Piludu, M. A, Lober, S., Hubner, H., Gmeiner, P., Argiolas, A., Giorgi, O., (2013). Dopamine agonist-induced penile erection and yawning: a comparative study in outbred Roman high- and low-avoidance rats. *Pharmacol. Biochem. Behav.* 109, 59-66. doi: 10.1016/j.pbb.2013.05.002.
6. SANNA, F., Ortner, B., Hübner, H., Löber, S., Tschammer, N., Gmeiner, P., (2013). Discovery of dopamine D(4) receptor antagonists with planar chirality. *Bioorg. Med. Chem.*. 21, 1680-1684. doi: 10.1016/j.bmc.2013.01.065.
7. SANNA, F., Melis, M. R., Angioni, L., Argiolas, A., (2013). Clavulanic acid induces penile erection and yawning in male rats: Comparison with apomorphine. *Pharmacol. Biochem. Behav.*. 103, 750-755. doi: 10.1016/j.pbb.2012.12.001.
8. Löber, S., Hübner, H., Buschauer, A., SANNA, F., Argiolas, A., Melis, M. R., Gmeiner, P., (2012). Novel Azulene Derivatives for the Treatment of Erectile Dysfunction. *Bioorg. Med. Chem. Lett.* 22,, 7151-7154. doi: 10.1016/j.bmcl.2012.09.064.
9. SANNA, F., Argiolas, A., Melis, M. R., (2012). Oxytocin-induced yawning: sites of action in the brain and interaction with mesolimbic/mesocortical and incertohypothalamic dopaminergic neurons in male rats. *Horm. Behav.*. 62, 505-514. doi: 10.1016/j.yhbeh.2012.08.010.
10. Melis, M.R., SANNA, F., Succu, S., Ferri, G. L., Argiolas, A., (2012). Neuroendocrine Regulatory Peptide-1 and Neuroendocrine Regulatory Peptide-2 influence differentially feeding and penile erection in male rats: sites of action in the brain. *Reg. Pept.* 177, 46-52. doi: 10.1016/j.regpep.2012.04.007.

11. SANNA, F., Succu, S., Melis, M. R., Argiolas, A., (2012). Dopamine agonists induced penile erection and yawning: differential role of D2-like receptor subtypes and correlation with nitric oxide production in the paraventricular nucleus of the hypothalamus of male rats. *Behav. Brain Res.* 230, 355-364. doi: 10.1016/j.bbr.2012.02.033.
12. SANNA, F., Succu, S., Hübner, H., Gmeiner, P., Argiolas, A., Melis. M. R., (2011). Dopamine D2-like receptor agonists induce penile erection in male rats: differential role of D2, D3 and D4 receptors in the paraventricular nucleus of the hypothalamus. *Behav. Brain Res.* 225, 169-176. doi: 10.1016/j.bbr.2011.07.018.

INDEX

D

E

F

G

H

I

K

L

M

N

S

T

U

V

W